Praise for *Around*
and Rosan

"Rosanne Bane understands not only the resistance all writers face but the neurological basis of that resistance. Her ingenious application of research about our brains to the process of writing and her wise counsel overall can help writers at every level."

—RALPH KEYES, AUTHOR OF *THE COURAGE TO WRITE* AND *THE WRITER'S BOOK OF HOPE*

"Compared to the ubiquitous 'inspirational' artists' guides that seem determined to free your inner child and invite angels to perch on your shoulder, the approach taken by Rosanne Bane in *Around the Writer's Block* strikes me as singularly refreshing and intelligent. Bane introduces the many obstacles commonly lumped under the heading of 'writer's block' by providing detailed descriptions of how different parts of the brain connect and interact when faced with different mental challenges—and then uses that knowledge to fashion responses artists can use to good advantage as they set about trying to get at the writing they need to do."

—TED ORLAND, COAUTHOR OF *ART & FEAR*

"*Around the Writer's Block* gives writers the tools we need to tackle the resistance born inside our own brains. And the best part? You don't have to be a brain surgeon to put Rosanne Bane's practical and profound advice to immediate use in accelerating toward your own writing goals!"

—LISA BULLARD, IRA/CBC CHILDREN'S CHOICE AWARD–WINNING AUTHOR OF *TRICK-OR-TREAT ON MILTON STREET* AND *NOT ENOUGH BEDS*

"Rosanne Bane's compassion for writers struggling with writer's block (and more subtle forms of resistance) combined with the ability to explain in clear, simple language how brain science applies to writers, make this book a gift to both aspiring and established writers. *Around the Writer's Block* gives writers everywhere the information, habits and tools they need to work through writing resistance."

—BRIAN MALLOY, AUTHOR OF *THE YEAR OF ICE, BRENDAN WOLF,* AND *TWELVE LONG MONTHS*

B + T

"Rosanne Bane's *Around the Writer's Block* was a book I could only read in short bursts because it so inspired me to get off my butt and write that I had to set the book down and tackle my own creative projects instead!"

—Tate Hallaway, bestselling author of
Tall, Dark & Dead

"Practical and energizing, Rosanne Bane's valuable exercises and healthy habits can successfully retrain your brain and creative spirit to manifest the dream that's in your heart."

—Mary Carroll Moore, award-winning author
of *Your Book Starts Here: Create, Craft, and Sell
Your First Novel, Memoir, or Nonfiction Book*

"Rosanne Bane has addressed all the excuses that keep us writers from producing."

—Pierce J. Howard, Ph.D., Managing Director of Research
and Development for the Center for Applied Cognitive
Studies and author of *The Owner's Manual for the Brain*

AROUND THE
WRITER'S BLOCK

JEREMY P. TARCHER/PENGUIN

a member of Penguin Group (USA) Inc.   New York

AROUND THE WRITER'S BLOCK

Using Brain Science to Solve Writer's Resistance*

*Including Writer's Block, Procrastination, Paralysis, Perfectionism, Postponing, Distractions, Self-Sabotage, Excessive Criticism, Overscheduling, and Endlessly Delaying Your Writing

Rosanne Bane

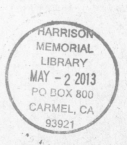

JEREMY P. TARCHER/PENGUIN
Published by the Penguin Group
Penguin Group (USA) Inc., 375 Hudson Street, New York, New York 10014, USA •
Penguin Group (Canada), 90 Eglinton Avenue East, Suite 700, Toronto, Ontario M4P 2Y3,
Canada (a division of Pearson Penguin Canada Inc.) • Penguin Books Ltd,
80 Strand, London WC2R 0RL, England • Penguin Ireland, 25 St Stephen's Green,
Dublin 2, Ireland (a division of Penguin Books Ltd) • Penguin Group (Australia),
250 Camberwell Road, Camberwell, Victoria 3124, Australia (a division of Pearson
Australia Group Pty Ltd) • Penguin Books India Pvt Ltd, 11 Community Centre,
Panchsheel Park, New Delhi–110 017, India • Penguin Group (NZ), 67 Apollo Drive,
Rosedale, North Shore 0632, New Zealand (a division of Pearson New Zealand Ltd) •
Penguin Books (South Africa) (Pty) Ltd, 24 Sturdee Avenue, Rosebank, Johannesburg 2196,
South Africa

Penguin Books Ltd, Registered Offices: 80 Strand, London WC2R 0RL, England

"Synaptic Jazz"© 2012 by Jean Cook. Reprinted with permission from author.

Most Tarcher/Penguin books are available at special quantity discounts for bulk purchase
for sales promotions, premiums, fund-raising, and educational needs. Special books
or book excerpts also can be created to fit specific needs. For details, write
Penguin Group (USA) Inc. Special Markets, 375 Hudson Street, New York, NY 10014.

ISBN 978-1-58542-871-7

Printed in the United States of America
10 9 8 7 6 5 4 3 2 1

BOOK DESIGN BY MEIGHAN CAVANAUGH

While the author has made every effort to provide accurate telephone numbers
and Internet addresses at the time of publication, neither the publisher nor the
author assumes any responsibility for errors, or for changes that occur after
publication. Further, the publisher does not have any control over and does not
assume any responsibility for author or third-party websites or their content.

Synaptic Jazz

by Jean Cook

Each neuron
in your head
aims to stop dead
your saboteur.

Ganglia thick like
Medusa's snake hair
their dendrites lively, aware
aquiver, writhing,
release, receive enzymes
time and again and time
firing with willpower
every minute, every hour
firing, conspiring,
aspiring to inspire to aspire.

Never flogging your noggin,
snap-crackle-pop,
your impulses don't stop
rapid fire rat-a-tat-tat

whadya think about that?
about this?
snapping across the synapse gaps
across the abyss
nerves with verve and flair
analyze, improvise
how to get from here to there,
from there to here?
Brain smiles and waves
staves off the fear
strolling la-di-da
past the amygdala.

A shower of brainpower
lightning paths cutting swaths
across your gray matter
connecting a smattering
of what's mattering,
of this, of that,
so much going on under your hat
brimming full
of natural chemicals
of dopamine,
know what I mean?
Brainstorms
are the norm.

Your methodical plotting
not plodding
around the writer's block

steady as a rock
steady as you go
the ideas flow
axon to axon, flow on
past snake brain
the electron convoy conveys
an energy load along vertabrae
neverendin' at the tendons
now going far
going intramuscular
through bicep, tricep,
funnels into the carpal tunnel
through your finger,
through your pen
and then
ideas swirl
into the world.

Creativity,
It's cerebral, baby.

CONTENTS

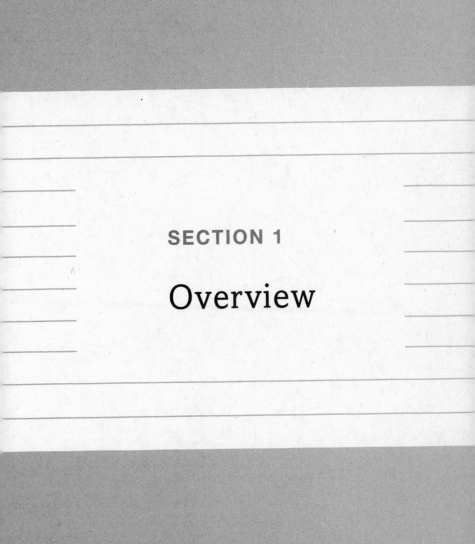

SECTION 1

Overview

1

INTRODUCTION

What Do They Got That I Ain't Got?

Some people seem able to write no matter what's going on: work stress, a flood of family activities and responsibilities, health issues, a string of rejection letters, a furnace that quits in Minnesota in February. Do these people have more willpower than the rest of us? More discipline? Are they less susceptible to distractions? Or just more self-centered?

The students and coaching clients I work with aren't more disciplined, focused or self-focused than most people. But they show up for their writing and themselves because they've learned how to harness the power of habit. They've learned what's going on in their brains when they're feeling resistance, and what they can do to move through that resistance. I give them encouragement, information and tools to figure out how to make writing part of their lives, but the truth is, they're the ones who show up and do the work. They've helped me refine my coaching and hone the basic practices that create sustainable habits. I thank and applaud them all! You'll want to thank them too when you learn what they know about fighting resistance and showing up for your writing.

This book is for all of us who love to write and yet avoid our writing at least some of the time. It's for all of us who:

- Want to write, but can't figure out where to start or what to say.
- Promise ourselves we'll write "someday" and miss opportunities to write right now.
- Find our home gets cleaner and cleaner the closer we come to a deadline.
- Edit our first page over and over and feel unable or unworthy to move on.
- Keep our schedules so full we don't have time to write.
- Take care of everyone else before writing.
- Suddenly remember ten other things that require immediate attention when we sit down to write.
- Procrastinate and delay our dreams.
- Delay or fail to meet deadlines.
- Play it safe and avoid the risk of being fully present and vulnerable on the page.
- Give all our time to writing projects that neither challenge nor excite us.
- Sabotage our own efforts with lost files, accidents or missed appointments.

We sit down in our writing space, only to pop out of the chair to get a drink, a snack, another book to research. Or we sit down at our computers to write, but first we have to check and respond to email and somehow an hour goes by and we never quite got to the writing. Or we never quite make our way to the writing space at all. We distract ourselves with a multitude of other things to do and think about. We keep promising ourselves that someday soon we'll go back to the novel, the poems, the essay about Great-aunt Ruby. And while we're promising ourselves we'll return to what gives us such joy, some small part of us knows that we're lying.

Why do we have such a love-fear relationship with our writing? What is it about writing that both attracts and repels us? Why is it so difficult to do the very thing we love?

Resistance Is Normal

Fortunately, not every writer is going to experience the paralysis of full-blown writer's block, but every writer experiences some kind of resistance from time to time. It doesn't matter whether you're writing for your career, to finish a degree, or for personal satisfaction. It's doesn't matter whether you've published for years or you're still looking for your first publishing credit. What matters is not whether you will face resistance, but how you'll face it.

Resistance shows up in many different ways. Some writers get anxious—and let's face it, there's plenty to get nervous about: being rejected, rejecting yourself, harsh criticism, offending people, indifference, not being able to write, not being able to write anything worthwhile, not writing well and not knowing it until you've made a fool of yourself in public. Sometimes we're aware of the fear and how it keeps us from our writing; other times, we don't recognize that it's fear that is making us so susceptible to distractions despite our desire to write.

Some writers get nasty—horribly critical of themselves and others, and openly mean in expressing that criticism. Some writers get busy—distracting themselves from the underlying fear by keeping themselves too busy to write. Some writers get tired—falling on a spectrum that runs from giving in to the sudden overwhelming need for a nap to chronic fatigue to clinical depression. Some of us get rebellious—"Who do I think I am, telling me what to do?" Some of us get wimpy and vague—"Of course I'll write. About something. Sometime. But first . . ."

For many of us, resistance is a shape-changer, shifting from one form to another. Just when we start to realize what's going on, the resistance finds a new form.

All of this is normal. It's not comfortable, but it is normal. Resistance is part of the writing life. What makes or breaks us is not whether or how we experience resistance—it's how we respond to resistance. Most writers respond badly: we criticize ourselves; we push and drive; we threaten and bully ourselves; we question our ability, our commitment, our character. We must stop doing this! It is completely ineffective. It drains the joy out of writing. And sometimes, in the worst-case scenarios, the resistance wins out, and someone who could have been a good writer gives up on writing altogether.

Resistance Can Be Resolved

Resistance is not about laziness, lack of willpower, or the failure of intellect and imagination. It's about neurology and psychology. And when we know what's happening in our brain when we feel resistant, we can learn how to respond effectively.

The best response is to write around the resistance. We need simple practices that bring us to our writing space regularly. We need commitments that are meaningful enough to engage us and small enough to give us confidence that we can keep showing up no matter what.

Around the Writer's Block will give you the information, encouragement and pragmatic tools you need to move through resistance and get your ideas on the page and into the world. This book explains, in easy-to-understand language, our best understanding of what's going on in a writer's brain when she/he experiences resistance. It combines the insights of recent neurological research with my twenty years of experience in teaching creativity, coaching creative people, and studying the creative process.

As a teacher and coach, I've challenged and encouraged thousands of novelists, short-story writers, playwrights, poets, memoirists, nonfiction writers, songwriters, storytellers, bloggers, graduate students, and business writers to share their unique perspective with a variety of audiences. I continue to talk with writers across the country about how resistance has affected their writing, how they've tried to overcome resistance, and what actually works for them.

I'm going to give you proven practices and methods that I've seen work for my students, coaching clients and colleagues, including established professional writers, aspiring and emerging writers, and people who need to write well in academia and business. These practices will work for you, too.

CHALLENGE: RESISTANCE INVENTORY

My coaching clients determine what projects they want to work on, what goals they want to achieve and what action steps they'll take to get there. They set the agenda, but occasionally I'll suggest a challenge to them. Challenges can be accepted, modified or declined altogether. I offer challenges rather than "homework" or "exercises" to honor my clients' commitment and autonomy. I'll do the same for you. Throughout this book, you'll find challenges, which you can accept as is, modify to better suit your situation, or decline altogether.

If you want to decline a challenge because it simply doesn't interest you or apply to you, that's fine. But if a challenge intrigues you, and especially if it disturbs you, respond to it right then using whatever tools are available. If you find that all the challenges seem boring or irrelevant, consider the possibility that this might be a form of resistance and push yourself to do the challenges, particularly the ones that "bore" you the most or seem the "least relevant."

You'll often freewrite your responses to challenges. If you are not familiar with the term (coined by Natalie Goldberg in *Writing Down the Bones*), don't worry. Freewriting is writing nonstop without judgment, editing or second-guessing yourself. Whatever comes into your head goes on the page. Don't worry about how it sounds or whether you're using the best word. Don't worry about spelling, punctuation, making complete sentences or even making complete sense. Just keep your hand moving, even if you have to repeat yourself or write, "I don't know what to write," over and over or make stuff up. Set a timer for ten minutes and just keep your hand moving until time's up. And if you want to keep writing when the timer goes off, by all means, go for it.

By the way, it doesn't really matter what you use to respond to these challenges. If you keep a writer's journal, you can write your responses there. Or you can collect responses to the challenges in a computer folder, a notebook, a three-ring binder, or leave them scattered wherever they fall. It doesn't even matter whether you keep your responses to the challenges; feel free to recycle them as soon as you finish them if you like. The important thing is doing at least some of the challenges.

Whatever you do, don't use the lack of an "official challenge journal" as the reason you tell yourself, "I can't do this now. I'll just skip over this now and come back later." Because in all likelihood, you won't return, and keeping the promises you make to yourself is crucial in establishing the kind of habits that will support your writing.

Here's your first challenge:

Step 1: Freewrite for ten minutes about what resistance has cost you as a writer and what it has cost your community. What opportunities have you lost? What dreams have you delayed? What stories have you left untold; what images and insights have you left unshared? What problems could your writing help solve?

Step 2: Freewrite for ten minutes about what you truly want to do with your writing energy and time.

What are you willing to do to resolve your resistance so you can start doing what you really want to do?

The Power of a Writing Habit

For more than ten of the twenty years I've instructed writers on the creative process at the Loft Literary Center in Minneapolis (the country's largest and most comprehensive independent literary center), I have taught a class called The Writing Habit. For many, this is their first Loft class, their first experience with writers teaching writers, and their first bold claim that maybe they are writers, too.

Other students turn to The Writing Habit after taking several craft-focused classes at the Loft in fiction, creative nonfiction, poetry or other genres. Some have MFAs or advanced degrees in writing or literature. Some are trying to complete their dissertation. Some are or have been professional writers who discover that they're great at meeting deadlines their bosses and editors set, but they need a different kind of structure to keep them accountable when they're working on projects that don't have deadlines yet.

One of the common things I hear from my Loft students is a bemused confession that, even though they love to write, they seem to have an unending supply of excuses for not writing what they really want to. They are shocked by how much time has passed since they wrote consistently, or surprised they aren't writing regularly even though it's been months since they've finished what they thought was delaying their writing—earning their master's degree, getting the kids out of diapers, getting the kids off to college, completing a major project at work, retiring.

That's where we start: with the awareness that their current methods aren't working. I promise my students they can have a sustainable and satisfying writing practice based on three basic habits—Process, Product Time (a.k.a. writing time) and Self-care—and that these three habits will make it possible to show up for their writing. Then, and only then, can they return to the joy and satisfaction that comes from doing what they love to do. It's still difficult at times, because resistance is omnipresent, but they know how to show up and write in spite of the resistance.

If you want more joy, consistency and productivity in your writing life, I promise you that you too can discover how to build the habits that allow you write your way around your writer's block.

INSIDE THE WRITER'S BRAIN: NEURAL PATHWAYS

A habit is a neural pathway in the brain. Neurons that are stimulated more often grow a thicker layer of myelin, which insulates neurons. The thicker the myelin sheath around the neurons in a particular pathway, the faster and more accurately the signals along that pathway travel. The more a behavior or thought pattern is repeated, the more efficient the neural pathway for that behavior or thought becomes. A habit is nothing more than a well-myelinated neural pathway.[1]

WRITER'S APPLICATION: GETTING OUT OF THE RUT

Back when I was in college, I hiked part of the Appalachian Trail. There were sections of the trail so overused that the ruts were just a little wider than a hiking boot and nearly knee-deep. Because these ruts were so deep and narrow, it was difficult, even painful, to walk in them. But given the nature of the trail in those spots, there was little choice. The repetition of hiking boots falling in the same places made the ruts deeper and narrower as the years passed.

This is what bad habits are: neural pathways that are so well traveled, it is extremely difficult to get out of the rut no matter how painful it is to repeat the old behavior.

As we'll explore in more depth in chapter two, the good news is that the brain is highly plastic—that is, capable of significant change, not just in childhood, but throughout our entire life. Behavior is both determined by brain activity and the determiner of brain activity. That means that we can learn new habits, and, as we myelinate new neural pathways, the old habits fade.

INQUIRY

If I were your creativity coach, I'd give you a different open-ended question to ponder at the end of each coaching session. In this book, I will give you an inquiry at the end of each chapter that reflects the issues the chapter is likely to raise for you. These inquiries acknowledge that you know your writing practices and life better than anyone else, and are designed to encourage you to own the information and the change process you're embarking on.

Here's your first inquiry: "If I could wake up tomorrow with any habit I want ingrained in my brain and my behavior—without the effort of practicing daily for many weeks to develop that habit—what habit would I want?"

2

WHY IS IT SO HARD TO WRITE?

Why Do We Do That?

Why do we sit down in our writing space, only to pop out of the chair to look for answers in the refrigerator, empty the dishwasher, check the mail, or get another book to use for research?

Why do we have great ideas when we're in the shower or driving on the freeway, then freeze and not know how to start when we get to our writing space?

Why do we distract ourselves with a multitude of other things to do and think about?

Why do we paralyze ourselves with self-criticism and perfectionism?

Why is it so damned hard to write?

If I Only Had a Brain

The reason so many of us are left asking, "Why?" is because we don't have a brain—we have a *brain system*.

Just as the digestive system consists of separate organs with different jobs that work together to make it possible for the body to digest food, process nutrients and get rid of the excess, the brain consists of separate areas, each performing a separate, distinct purpose.

As noted neurologist Joseph LeDoux points out in *The Emotional Brain*, "Although we often talk about the brain as if it has a function, the brain itself actually has no function. It is a collection of systems, sometimes called modules, each with different functions."[1]

The separate yet integrated areas that make up the brain—the cortex, the thalamus, the cingulate system, the amygdala, and so on—are intricately connected and coordinated through a complex circuitry of neurons and an intricate dance of electrochemical activity. The various components of the brain collaborate to achieve amazing feats, all the way from keeping the lungs breathing and the heart beating to the miracle that is consciousness: using language, making plans, knowing who we are, imagining we are someone else, choosing actions according to our moral code, and struggling with the knowledge of our own mortality.

But even with the profound collaboration among brain components, there are times when different parts of the brain compete. It is the potential conflict between the limbic system and the cerebral cortex that is most relevant to questions about our writing.

Brain Basics

Scientists typically identify three major systems of the human brain:

- The brain stem, or "lizard brain," which is located at the core of the entire brain system and maintains body functions like respiration, digestion and circulation.

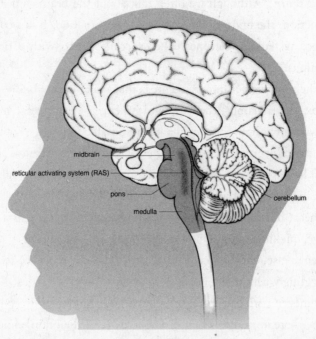

midbrain

reticular activating system (RAS)

pons

medulla

cerebellum

BRAIN STEM
© 2011 medicalartstudio.com

- The limbic system, or "leopard brain," which surrounds the brain stem and provides the capacity for emotion and relies on the fight-or-flight instinct in response to threats.

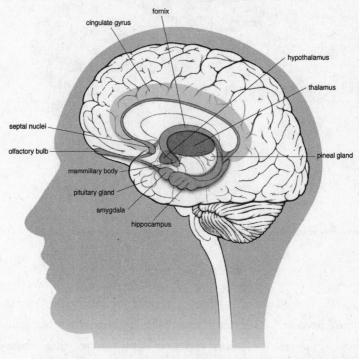

LIMBIC SYSTEM
© 2011 *medicalartstudio.com*

- The cerebral cortex, or "learning brain," which surrounds the limbic system and gives us the ability to solve problems, use language and numbers, create, anticipate the future, motivate ourselves, and reflect on and modify our behavior.[2,3]

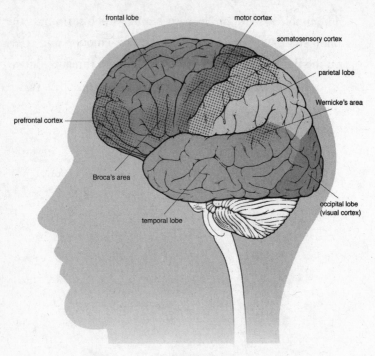

CORTEX
© 2011 medicalartstudio.com

The human limbic system is sometimes called the "leopard brain" because it is very similar to the limbic system in other mammals. It processes sensory experiences and passes that sensory information to the cortex. But the limbic system also gives emotion to our sensory experiences so that by the time that sensory information is perceived by the cortex, the information has an emotional association. The limbic system is made up of the thalamus, hypothalamus, pituitary gland, hippocampus, pineal gland, mammillary body, fornix, cingulate gyrus and, as we'll see later in this chapter, the star of the limbic show: the amygdala.

The human cortex, particularly the prefrontal cortex, is significantly different from the cortices of other mammals. This "learning brain" makes humans truly human. The cortex consists of four lobes: the frontal lobe (a.k.a. the "executive lobe," which conceptualizes, forms goals, devises plans, motivates behavior, and evaluates results and the appropriateness of behavior), the temporal lobe (which processes sound, comprehends speech and handles some aspects of learning and memory), the occipital lobe (which processes vision), and the parietal lobe (which integrates all sensory information, controls movement and orientation, and calculates and handles some aspects of recognition). Within each lobe, there are areas that have particular functions. For example, Broca's area is central in producing language, while Wernicke's area is responsible for comprehending language.

The brain stem is composed of the cerebellum, midbrain, pons, medulla, and the reticular activating system (RAS), which monitors information coming in from the senses and filters what you pay attention to and what you ignore. For example, in a crowded room, you can't hear what someone ten feet away is saying, but if that person says your name, your RAS makes sure you hear it.

Who's Driving the Bus?

If you're not used to thinking of your brain as a collection of these three major systems, you might think of your brain as the driver and your body as the vehicle. You might even think of your brain as a highly skilled driver capable of split-second decisions and lightning-fast reactions, in total command of the Ferrari race car that is your body. But a better metaphor would be to see your body as a bus and your brain as a group of drivers, all jostling for the opportunity to get behind the wheel.

Your cortex is the driver who cares about writing and has the "executive functions" needed to write: imagining the future, envisioning possible outcomes, setting goals, making plans, and motivating and monitoring your own behavior. As long as your cortex is driving the bus, you'll care about your commitments to write and take action to fulfill your writing goals.

But your cortex isn't the only driver. The reticular activating system not only filters what you pay attention to, it also serves as a kind of toggle switch that determines who's driving the bus: the limbic system or the cortex. When we relax, the RAS flips control to the cortex and we are capable of the symbolic, logical and creative thinking that is the hallmark of human evolution. When the cortex is behind the wheel, we're able to focus our attention on and take action to support our creative aspirations.

Limbic System Takeovers

But when we perceive a potential threat, the RAS flips control to the limbic system and we rely on our instinctual fight-or-flight response. The amygdala is engaged and triggers the release of stress hormones like cortisol and adrenaline. Heart rate increases, vision tunnels, the palms sweat, the hair on the back of the neck stands up, blood moves from the torso to the large muscles in the extremities to allow fast movement. In this state, our emotional reactions are intense and we can say and do things that we will later regret. Road rage is one result of a limbic system takeover; the brain-freeze of being unable to think of a response to a rude person until that person is long gone is another; and jumping back or running away from a spider or a snarling dog is another. When the limbic system takes over, creativity is dismissed as trivial compared to the need to take immediate action to stay alive and safe.

When the limbic system has been activated, we react automatically from instinct or training. Combat soldiers endure intense training and airplane pilots practice emergency maneuvers in flight simulators so that their training will override their instincts when their limbic systems are activated.

With the limbic system driving the bus, the cortex is effectively shut down. We are still conscious—we can still speak and calculate—so we often don't know that the cortex has been elbowed out of the driver's seat, but what we say and how we act are based on previous training. We are not capable of innovative, nuanced thinking, and our choices in this state will be instinctive. None of the higher thinking functions—the frontal cortex's "executive functions"—are available.

Unfortunately, your cortex doesn't do a particularly good job of recognizing when it's been pushed out of the driver's seat. Imagine a driver sitting in a passenger seat on a bus with a Playskool dashboard on her or his lap, moving the toy wheel and pushing toy brakes and getting frustrated and confused when the bus doesn't turn and move the way the driver wants. That's about what happens when the limbic system is in control and the cortex doesn't recognize that reality.

Consequently, we are literally of two minds about our creative work, depending on who's driving the bus. Our cortex seeks novelty and wants to be creative. The limbic system cares only about being safe and staying alive. When the limbic system is in control, we respond instinctively with behaviors that later make us shake our heads and say, "Now, why did I do that?"

We're often confused and sometimes embarrassed, frustrated, or remorseful about the actions we take when the limbic system is driving the bus. The cortex can't explain behavior initiated by the limbic system. Because the cortex doesn't recognize or accept that it wasn't in control, it makes up stories to try to explain what happened. Those stories include, "I'm lazy"; "I'm undisciplined"; "Maybe I don't really want to write"; "Maybe I'm afraid of success." Or, as we'll see below, "I saw a snake and decided I should get away."

CHALLENGE: WHY DID I DO THAT?

List ten things you do that make you later wonder, "Why did I do that?" Set judgment aside as you're making the list. Let yourself be in a state of genuine wonder, not regret or criticism.

INSIDE THE WRITER'S BRAIN: YOU CAN'T THINK BEFORE YOU JUMP

In *The Emotional Brain*, Dr. Joseph LeDoux explains how the cortex is often unaware that control has shifted.[4] For example, if you see a snake, you'll later say something like, "I saw a snake and thought I should get away, so I jumped." However, the faster limbic system made your body jump *before* your cortex had the conscious thought, "I should jump."

More specifically, the visual stimulus is first processed by the visual thalamus, which sends crude information—in this case, "snakelike object"—to the amygdala. The amygdala kicks the body into the fight-or-flight mode described above. In the case of seeing what might be a snake, the amygdala sends impulses down the spinal column to the nerves that make us jump out of the way.

The visual thalamus also sends information to the visual cortex, which makes finer distinctions (e.g., "Is this in fact a snake or just a stick?"). The visual cortex sends this refined information to the amygdala, but by this time, we've already jumped. Only after we've jumped to safety does the amygdala bring the cortex into the decision-making loop. Incredible egotist that the cortex is, we all think, "I saw a snake and I thought I'd better get out of the way, so I jumped," despite the fact that we jumped *before* we had the conscious awareness of the need to jump.

In other words, the cortex fails to recognize when it's not driving the bus.

Meet Aimee

You can meet Aimee, but Aimee can't meet you. Of course, you can't really meet a person in a book, but even if you were to appear at the Asile de Bel-Air hospital in France in 1906, where

Aimee (not her real name) was a patient of Dr. Edouard Claparède, and shook Aimee's hand, she would not be able to truly meet you.

As a result of a brain injury, Aimee lost the ability to form new memories. While her memories of her life before the injury were unimpaired, after she was injured, Aimee couldn't remember anything that happened more than a few minutes earlier.

So every time Dr. Claparède saw Aimee, he had to introduce himself as if he were meeting her for the first time. Claparède decided to conduct a small experiment one day. He put a pin between the fingers of his right hand, so that when he walked into the room, introduced himself, and shook hands with Aimee, she received a surprising, painful, but harmless stab in the palm of her hand. Claparède apologized and talked with her for a few minutes, then left. Aimee, of course, had no memory of the incident.[5]

And yet, when Claparède reached for Aimee's hand when "meeting" her later, she pulled her hand away. She refused to shake hands with him, even though she had never refused to do so before, and even though she couldn't explain why she was unwilling to shake his hand.

Aimee's resistance to shaking Claparède's hand makes perfect sense to us. But keep in mind that Aimee could not retain new memories. She didn't remember the pin, so she couldn't explain her resistance. Aimee's experience demonstrates that memories, especially memories of painful experiences, are laid down in the brain with at least two systems. Aimee had lost the ability to form new conscious memories, but apparently her unconscious memory system still functioned well enough for her to avoid the threat of shaking Claparède's hand.

Claparède couldn't adequately explain Aimee's memory failure or how she managed to retain enough "memory" to know not to shake his hand. In *The Emotional Brain*, Joseph LeDoux elaborates, "It now seems that Claparède was seeing the operation of two different memory systems in his patient—one involved in forming memories of experience and making those memories available for conscious recollection at some later time, and another operating outside of consciousness and controlling behavior without explicit awareness of the past learning."[6]

The key point of Aimee's story is that you don't have to have a conscious memory or a "logical" reason for feeling resistant. And just because you don't know why you don't want to do something doesn't mean there isn't a good reason for not doing it.

As LeDoux puts it, "Although the patient did not have a conscious memory of the situation, subconsciously she learned that shaking Claparède's hand could cause her harm, and her brain used this stored information, this memory, to prevent the unpleasantness from occurring again."[7]

Who's Your Dr. Claparède?

You've undoubtedly gotten reactions to your writing that were far more unpleasant than a little pinprick. It doesn't matter whether it was your third-grade teacher marking your punctuation errors in thick red pencil, a poisonous TA ridiculing your poetry in sophomore English, or some relative urging you to "stop that silly scribbling and live up to your potential."

You might expect a challenge here to list the people and situations that have embarrassed or pained you about your writing. But there really isn't much point in looking for causes; there are far too many possibilities and nothing to be gained from inventorying past injuries.

It is enough to know that when you feel resistance, there is a legitimate reason for it. Interestingly, when Aimee was pushed to explain why she wouldn't shake Claparède's hand, she said something like, "Doesn't one have the right to withdraw her hand?"[8] In other words, her cortex, unable to explain her reservations, made something up. Remember that the cortex does a poor job of recognizing when it's not in control. Your cortex is probably busy making up stories to explain behavior prompted by your limbic system far more often than you realize.

Rather than admit we just don't know why we did something or why we don't want to do something—a profound statement of vulnerability few of us are capable of—we rationalize, make assumptions, and draw erroneous conclusions from inadequate evidence. Writers often assume the worst: that we're lazy, undisciplined or lack willpower, intelligence and ambition. Or we complain about writer's block. Or we distract ourselves and fill our schedules with other priorities to give us the illusion of virtue and allow us to claim a reason, any reason, not to write. "I'm too busy to write. Maybe after I . . ."

Unfortunately, none of these responses helps us get past the resistance caused by the limbic system's takeover. In fact, negative assumptions and rationalizations often make us more stressed, and stress only increases the need to keep the limbic system in control. Unchecked and misinterpreted, resistance can lead to an ongoing cycle where the anxiety of anticipating not being able to write triggers the limbic system and reinforces the resistance. At an extreme, we call this self-perpetuating cycle "writer's block."

You are not being weak willed, thin-skinned, oversensitive, underdisciplined, or lazy. You are reacting to a subconscious awareness of a potential threat. In fact, your cortex is probably far more consistent about showing up for your writing than you give yourself credit for. That is, your cortex is consistent *when* it's in charge, which is less often than your cortex recognizes.

The relevant question is not, "Why am I behaving this way?" or, "Why am I so lazy?" (or some other harsh, judgmental word), but, "How can I respond to get what I really want: the freedom to enjoy writing and the power to write effectively?"

Writing Is Its Own Reward— or Threat

As marvelous as it feels to be in the flow, writing is more often a source of stress than bliss for all of us. You have an audience to please, a deadline to meet, an idea you want to share that refuses to be pinned down, not to mention the memories, conscious and unconscious, of all the criticism, correction and rejection your writing has received in the past. And if that's not enough, many of us fear success, because it means putting ourselves out there where we run the risks of exposing ourselves too much, being judged and criticized, or offending people we care about.

At least some of the time in writing and in life, you're going to feel frightened, anxious, angry or embarrassed. And when you do, your RAS will shift control to your limbic system. Your limbic system doesn't care about how much you're growing as a writer or how rewarding it will be to get your work appreciated or published. Its job is to keep you alive, and the best way to do that is to rely on the old tried-and-true instincts that have guided humans for millions of years. When your limbic system takes over—and it will—all the promises that "this time will be different" and "this time I'll really stick to my writing schedule" become irrelevant.

Since we all have had negative experiences around our writing, we often come to writing with our limbic systems triggered, even if we aren't aware of it. Or we avoid writing altogether because our limbic system is triggered, again without our conscious awareness. It is simply impossible to write well when the limbic system has precedence over the creative cortex.

Until we learn how to flip the RAS from limbic system to cortex, our efforts to be "disciplined" about our writing will be futile since none of the higher cognitive functions necessary for writing will be available. Learning just a little bit more about the neurological causes of resistance will help you recognize resistance in its many guises and find ways to relax so that your cortex can reengage.

Recognizing Resistance

The many forms of resistance can be categorized by the instinctive actions we take when the limbic system is triggered. When threatened, all mammals will freeze for a moment before choosing to fight or flee.

Freeze

This is usually a short-lived reaction. We typically freeze for a moment, then move into fighting or fleeing. When this "deer in the headlights" response is repeated for more than a few days, we traditionally call it "writer's block." Because the RAS has flipped control to the limbic system, the innovative and sophisticated thinking of the frontal cortex is not available. The writer literally cannot think what to write or how to start. The prolonged freeze response can cause emotional numbness or intense anxiety and frustration.

Fight

The fight response can be directed at yourself, at someone else, or both. Fighting yourself includes excessively harsh criticism, negative self-talk, hating the writing or yourself, perfectionism, and sabotage behaviors such as missing deadlines, losing files, having accidents, etc. Fighting others can include refusing to hear suggestions for revision, criticizing other writers or other people in your life, insisting that you're right or insisting on doing it your way, denying the need for improvement, damning the whole system (publishing, academia, business, etc.).

Flee

The behaviors that rise from the urge to escape the discomfort associated with writing are the most common forms of resistance. These include distractions (social life, work, family obligations, other creative endeavors, hobbies, and numbing activities like excessive gaming, shopping, drinking, TV watching); the inability to stay in the chair to write; inventing other tasks that must be completed first (emails, cleaning the desk, researching beyond what's necessary); overscheduling or overcommitting to other priorities that "must" be addressed before the writing; waiting until the last minute to start; and other forms of procrastination.

All forms of resistance are confusing and frustrating. We seem unable to honor our best intentions and efforts to be better writers. It helps to remember that we are struggling so much because our limbic system is in charge, which leaves us unable to use our cortex for nuanced thought, self-reflection or the ability to foresee future outcomes. And it helps to know that you can bring your cortex back online.

CHALLENGE: HOW DO YOU DO?

Answer these questions about how you do resistance.

- How do I do the freeze response, and what do I usually do after the freeze? Do I stare at the blank screen, then flee to check my email? Or is it that little pause when I think about writing and then decide I'll do that later after I . . . ?

- How many ways do I run away from writing? How do I distract myself? What do I tell myself I need to do before I can write? How do I keep myself too busy to write?
- How and who do I fight? Who do I criticize? What do I complain about? What feedback or advice have I rejected?

Hope Is Not Lost

The good news is that there is a lot you can do to identify and manage your responses so that you can write effectively. An important first step is to bring resistance out of the shadows. Talk openly about your resistance with other writers, reminding one another that this is not an excuse to avoid creative work, but an opportunity to devise and share strategies to overcome common forms of resistance.

The appendix will help you start your own Around the Writer's Block support group, or you can visit www.Facebook .com/AWBWritersGroups, to add yourself to the list of writers who are interested in supporting each other in recognizing and resolving writer's resistance.

The remaining chapters of *Around the Writer's Block* will detail what else you need to know and what you can do to bring ease and joy to your writing life.

Plastic Brain to the Rescue!

The best news is that the human brain "is wired for change," says Dr. Ira Black, professor and chair of the Department of Neuroscience and Cell Biology at the Robert Wood Johnson Medical School.[9]

The concept of neuroplasticity, the idea that the brain can change far more than we ever thought possible, is probably one of the landmark shifts in science, up there with Einstein's rewriting the laws of physics or Copernicus disproving the Church's decree that the sun circled the Earth. The old paradigm was that the human brain grew and developed in infancy and childhood, and that once we reached adulthood our brains would only decline because neurons could not be replaced. Adult brains were computing machines and, like machines, they were fixed, "hardwired." The brain couldn't alter its structure or change how it processed information.

Paradigms die hard, and in the 1970s, researchers who found evidence to challenge the old paradigm were not welcomed with open minds. They were ridiculed, accused of poor research methods and denied opportunities to publish their research findings. But the researchers persevered, the evidence piled higher, and now neuroplasticity is widely accepted.

We now know that the brain can grow new neurons and reorganize itself by making new neural connections to compensate for injury or to adjust to changes in the environment. Dr. Jill Bolte Taylor, author of *My Stroke of Insight*, explains neuroplasticity by comparing the brain to a playground filled with children playing different games in different places. If the kids can't play on the jungle gym, they don't just stop playing; they play with other kids on the swings or the slide. Likewise, neurons don't just hang around doing nothing when the function they were performing is no longer available.[10]

Not surprisingly, research has shown that blind people who read Braille have more neurons in the somatosensory cortex (which processes tactile sensations) dedicated to feeling in the finger they use to read than nonblind people or blind people who don't read Braille. What's amazing is that not only are they using the neurons in the somatosensory cortex to read Braille, they also use the neurons in the visual cortex. As Taylor suggests, the neurons in the visual cortex don't lie dormant; the visual cortex rewires itself so that those neurons are available for a different purpose. Even more amazing, neurons in the visual cortex not only adapt to "read" Braille, they also contribute to other language-processing tasks, something that is supposedly reserved for the nonsensory, higher-cognitive parts of the cortex.[11]

Like a corner lot in a thriving urban area, neurons are simply too valuable to leave unused for long.

Dr. Norman Doidge's *The Brain that Changes Itself* is a collection of incredible triumphs of neuroplasticity.[12] Doidge describes autistic children with dramatic increases in their abilities to use language and interact with others; blind people who are able to "see" words, faces, and shadows with a camera attached to eyeglasses that sends signals to an ultrathin strip of plastic on the tongue that in turn sends signals to the brain; and people in their eighties and nineties who were able to use physical and mental exercise to reverse the effects of aging on mood, memory, concentration and other cognitive abilities. These amazing stories may become commonplace as science expands our understanding of neuroplasticity.

We've long known that the brains of children are more plastic than those of adults, which may explain why children are more willing to engage in creative play and find it easier to learn all kinds of things, like a second language and figuring out how to use every function and app available on a smartphone (as any adult who's had to ask a child to decipher an electronic device can attest to). But we now know that the brain's ability to change persists throughout our lives. The brain is designed to keep learning, changing, and growing.

WRITER'S APPLICATION: YOU HAVE TO BE WILLING TO FAIL

Not only is the brain more plastic than we once thought, it is also more capable of healing than we once assumed. Stroke patients, for example, are more capable of recovering brain function than we realized was possible even as recently as ten years ago. Because we previously didn't think stroke victims could recover, they weren't encouraged to do what they needed to do to recover, and the belief became a self-fulfilling prophecy. A stroke kills neurons at the heart of the injury site. It also injures neurons surrounding the site of the stroke. As these surrounding neurons are repaired, the brain can recover some of its former ability. What's amazing is how much ability can be reclaimed and how contrary this reality is to what we once believed was possible. Dr. Edward Taub pioneered a treatment method that allowed people to regain the use of completely paralyzed hands, for example, that was successful even for patients who had their stroke years before treatment.[13]

The most important factor in recovering from a stroke is the patient's willingness to practice what she/he did effortlessly before the stroke.[14] If recovering neurons aren't challenged to do what they did before, they'll go work for some other function. If a stroke patient believes she/he can't recover use of her/his right hand, she/he won't practice using the right hand, and the belief becomes reality. Patients who refuse to give up, who face the frustration and keep practicing even when they're awkward and imperfect, are the ones who recover the most function.

I always tell my writing students that to write well, they have to write. And to write, they have to be willing to write badly. People who are willing to do something badly and keep practicing are the ones who improve; people who give up because they aren't willing to do it badly, don't.

As Malcolm Gladwell observes in *Outliers*, most so-called geniuses have logged at least 10,000 hours of practice before they "make it." What distinguishes the brilliant from the merely adequate is not "talent"; it's practice.[15]

CHALLENGE: RETRAIN YOUR BRAIN

Choose a physical activity you usually use your dominant hand for, like brushing your teeth or drawing or coloring, and practice doing it with your other hand. Or practice a simple activity you've never done before, like a specific series of ten dance steps. Allow yourself to do this activity badly. Don't worry about making mistakes, just practice. Record your progress for a week or so and notice how long it takes you to learn the new behavior and how long it takes for you to become proficient at it. Perfectionists think that insisting on near-perfect performance from the outset and criticizing themselves for every mistake will make them learn faster, but this actually impairs performance.

INQUIRY

"How many things have I given up in my life because it was too hard or I couldn't do it well enough? What do I love enough to be bad at?"

SECTION 2

Three Habits

*"Motivation is what gets you started.
Habit is what keeps you going."*

Jim Ryun

3

HABIT ONE: PROCESS

Success Story

Travel writer Ann Lonstein says, "I have been working on my habits for forty-five minutes a day and doing it! What helped me was to start each day with them, regardless of when I get up or what else I have to do. I do not drive myself crazy by setting alarms or working to a time commitment. I simply do them. I am also working on concentrating on doing only the task I am working on, not thinking, 'Oh, I should be doing this or that.' It has made a huge difference in what I get accomplished."

Ann is following an essential step in resolving resistance, one I give all my students and coaching clients: Make a little time on regular basis for the three habits of Process, Product Time (a.k.a. writing time) and Self-care. Practicing these three habits will give you profound results in your creativity.

These simple and flexible practices have a cumulative effect.

The more history you have with your habits, the more effect-ive they become for you. The longer you honor your commit-ments, the more momentum you have to carry you through tough times. I've seen this happen again and again with myself, my coaching clients and my students.

When I surveyed my current and former students and coaching clients, 338 established and aspiring writers responded. An addi-tional twenty writers who attended a convention where I spoke also responded. Eighty-eight percent of those who were familiar with the three habits I recommend reported that the practices reduced resistance. Eighty-seven percent reported that the prac-tices made it easier for them to face their resistance and still show up for their writing.

Process Time

The first of the three habits I encourage you to cultivate is Pro-cess. Process involves doing something fun that puts you in the creative flow. You do Process just for the sake of doing it; it's cre-ative play for play's sake. It's not about the outcomes—it's just about being in the creative flow on a regular basis. Practicing your ability to enter into the flow with a simple, regular Process activity of your choosing will increase your ability to draw on your creative power when you sit down to write.

When Julia Cameron urges readers of *The Artist's Way* and her other books to do morning pages (fill three pages in longhand every morning with strictly stream-of-consciousness writing), she's advising a type of Process. Process is also what Dorothea Brande is talking about when she encourages getting up early to "write easily and smoothly when the unconscious is in the ascendant" in *Becoming a Writer*.[1] Natalie Goldberg's freewriting, first introduced in *Writing Down the Bones*, is another form of Process.

When Brenda Ueland writes in *If You Want to Write*, "So you see the imagination needs moodling—long, inefficient, happy idling, dawdling and puttering," she's talking about the value of Process. She continues, "These people who are always briskly doing something and as busy as waltzing mice, they have little, sharp, staccato ideas. . . . But they have no slow, big ideas. And the fewer consoling, noble, shining, free, jovial, magnanimous ideas that come, the more nervously and desperately they rush and run from office to office and up and downstairs, thinking by action at last to make life have some warmth and meaning."[2] Amazingly, Ueland wrote that in 1938; what would she have to say about us today? We need the moodling found in Process more than ever.

Process can be morning pages or journaling, but there are many other options to choose from. Writers often benefit most from having a nonverbal Process practice. Here's a list of just some of things my clients, students, and I play with in our Process time:

- Keeping a dream journal
- Freewriting
- Listening to music
- Coloring in a coloring book
- Drawing mandalas
- Making collages

- Scrapbooking
- Sketching
- Painting (anything from finger painting to oil painting)
- Playing with clay or Play-Doh
- Taking photos
- Fooling around with an instrument
- Singing
- Daydreaming
- Dancing
- Knitting
- Watching people on the bus

Any kind of creative play that appeals to you, captures your focus, and allows you to get lost in the doing without fretting about the outcome is a good choice for Process. For example, listening fully and getting lost in music is Process, but half listening while you're busy doing something else is not.

INSIDE THE WRITER'S BRAIN: HANDS ON, BLOCK OFF

One hands-on solution to resistance is to literally get your hands off the keyboard and pick up a pen. According to *Newsweek*, "Brain scans show that handwriting engages more sections of the brain than typing."[3]

These aren't just any old sections of the brain being activated when you wield a pen. Virginia Berninger, professor of educational psychology at the University of Washington, refers to brain scans that show "sequential finger movements activated massive regions [of the brain] involved in thinking, language and working memory." These areas are essential for creative work and using a keyboard just doesn't engage them in the same way. Berninger points out that a keyboard allows you to select a whole letter with one touch, but handwriting "requires executing sequential strokes to form each letter."[4]

Another, even more hands-on solution is to back away, not just from the keyboard, but from words themselves, at least for a while. Borrowing from the storyboarding technique screenwriters use, Edwidge Danticat starts her novels with collages. After creating several collages, she uses "blue book" college exam notebooks to draft a novel before touching a computer keyboard. Danticat says "I like the tactile process. There's something old-fashioned about it, but what we do is kind of old-fashioned."[5]

Recent brain science explains why the old-fashioned tactile approach can be so effective. Sharon Begley observes "Although most of us think of motor skills and cognitive skills as like oil and water, in fact a number of studies have found that refining your sensory-motor skills can bolster cognitive ones. No one knows exactly why, but it may be that the two brain systems are more interconnected than we realize. So learn to knit, or listen to classical music, or master juggling, and you might be raising your IQ."[6, 7]

This may be one of the reasons Process is so effective in loosening up our creativity. This as-of-yet-unexplained connection between sensory-motor skills and cognitive abilities may explain why creative play breaks through mental blocks to deliver creative insight. Sometimes you need sensory-motor experiences that engage your body and fill your mind with images before you're ready to make words flow into sentences and paragraphs.

Follow Their Lead—or Create Your Own Dance

My coaching clients and students have a marvelous array of Process practices and receive an equally intriguing variety of benefits from their practices. Gordy Paquette, for example, relies on morning pages, which are for him "a form of prayer/meditation I address each day to my late grandmother and younger brother, Mark. Because so much of my writing involves the unfolding of memories, I turn to Grandma and Mark to help me sort out, face, love, and own all the parts of my life—and to honor them in the remembering. In return, I experience the morning pages as a sort of safe harbor where Grandma and Mark help me navigate the shoals at my day job where competing demands and office politics threaten my balance during the day."

Laura Sommers, copywriter and novelist, makes jewelry, gardens and sews for her Process. She observes, "I spend a lot of my time in a two-dimensional, black-and-white world, stringing together one word after another up in my head. So I follow these other creative pursuits purely because I love the doing of them. Today, before I wrote this, I hung several strings of glass beads I just bought in the window by my writing desk, just to catch the sunlight. I have a lot of writing work to get done today, but the beads will remind me to make time to play, too."

Stephanie Watson, author of *Elvis & Olive, Elvis & Olive: Super Detectives* and the upcoming picture book *The Wee Hours*, does comedy improv for her Process, which she performs every week in front of a live audience. "For someone who's used to creating and perfecting things in private, it's terrifying to make stuff up on the fly. Improv gives me the green light to be imperfect, embarrass myself, and take the emphasis off a polished product. Sometimes I am a big fool and fall flat on my face. Sometimes I am brilliant and get a big laugh. But it doesn't matter—either way, I walk away with the renewed ability to 'just go for it' in my art and in my life."

Sarah Tieck, editor, writing educator, and author of numerous published essays, articles, and children's nonfiction books, finds that Process is often a way to recharge her creative energy and fill the well. "With a full work schedule, I've got to be very intentional about Process—and flexible. Lately, I've been making elaborate and luscious meals. Sometimes I'll bake and decorate cupcakes. Other times, I garden, go to the movies, take photos, take a class, or try something new at the gym. When I write just for fun, I consider that Process, too. I've found that later, when I'm writing with more of a product focus, those just-for-fun pieces add glimmers of the unexpected into pieces that I otherwise might not be able to be as creative with. And when I've been doing a lot of creating and generating, there's something magical and satisfying about weeding my garden."

Surrender Expectations

Sarah Tieck highlights that some writing is clearly Process play, while other writing has "more of a product focus." So how do you know which is which and when you're truly doing Process? The essential difference is that you do Process with no expectations about the outcome. If you're journaling to discover a character's backstory, to identify the questions you need to address in an article, to explore issues you want to write about—in short, if you're writing something that will lead to writing you intend to publish or share in some other way, it's not Process. Those activities are what I call Product Time writing—that is, writing with a purpose in mind. We'll examine Product Time activities more closely in chapter four.

If something wonderful comes out of your Process time, that doesn't necessarily mean it's not Process. The important distinction is that when you're doing Process, making something might be a side effect, but it is not the goal. My friend Julie Theobald knits beautiful scarves, shawls, and baby blankets. Julie knits because the rhythm of her fingers repeating the same motion, the click of the needles and the repetition of reaching the end of the row and turning back again relaxes her and gives her quiet satisfaction. She sells or gives away most of what she knits so that she'll have the opportunity to choose another beautiful combination of yarn colors and textures and knit some more. The things she knits are the by-products; getting lost in the knitting is the real goal.

Process is about letting go of the demand that we need to

always be Doing Something Significant. It seems that we fear that if we stop doing something significant, we will stop being significant. We're so focused on *doing* constantly, we've forgotten how to just *be*. Process challenges us to surrender expectations and simply follow creative impulses without concern for the outcome. Process reminds us what we knew when we were kids—that it's easy to create when you stop worrying about what you're doing and just let the doing follow your being. The more often you access your creativity in Process when you don't need to care about outcomes (because they just don't matter in Process), the better prepared you'll be to direct that creativity during Product Time when you do care about the outcome.

Of course, playing around with Play-Doh for Process isn't going to improve your ability to handle dialogue or pacing. You have to practice those and other craft skills in your Product Time. But playing around with Play-Doh might open you up to new possibilities and make you more willing to experiment when you do tackle dialogue or pacing in your Product Time. Process helps us surrender the fears—of making mistakes or not knowing where we're going—that cause resistance.

One of the ways I do Process is to color in coloring books of mandalas and other geometric shapes. Coloring is fifteen minutes of freedom from the 201 things I have on my mind. It allows me to take a hiatus from "have to," "need to," and "should." When the biggest decision is whether to use the orange or green pencil next, and when there is no wrong choice because it doesn't matter what the end result looks like, my mental chatter diminishes and sometimes disappears altogether. As I surrender to the here and now of letting my imagination play in the present moment, I can hear the soft voice of my intuition again. Sometimes Process gives me new insights and ideas; it always gives me confidence and relaxation.

When your imagination is at play, you're in Process. When you let yourself just relax into the soft focus of play, where you are engaged without straining to concentrate, when you're active, but you're not pushing, you're in Process.

INSIDE THE WRITER'S BRAIN: A RIGHT-HEMISPHERE STATE OF MIND

Differences between the brain's left and right hemispheres are particularly relevant to creativity. Fortunately for us, Jill Bolte Taylor shares a unique and valuable perspective in her book *My Stroke of Insight*.[8] Dr. Taylor was a thirty-seven-year-old neuroanatomist working for the Harvard Brain Trust when a rare type of aneurysm burst in her brain, causing a severe stroke. *My Stroke of Insight* describes her amazing observations of remaining conscious while area after area of her left hemisphere shut down, leaving her unable to move the right half of her body, speak, comprehend how to use a telephone to call for help, and eventually to know who she was.

Taylor explains what it's like to have the normally dominant left hemisphere fall completely silent, how the right hemisphere perceives and interacts with the world, and how she integrated the two hemispheres as she made a remarkable eight-year recovery.

Many of Taylor's observations about hemispheric differences have been corroborated by research using SPECT brain imagery.

The left hemisphere is detail-focused and analytical; it compares and judges all things. The right hemisphere is focused on the whole, the big picture and similarities; it discerns differences without judgment. To the left hemisphere, time is measurable, divisible and sequential. But to the right hemisphere, time is fluid or unimportant; the right brain is always in the present moment in an unending here and now. While the right brain processes information slowly and, as Taylor says, "tends to hoe-de-doe along," the left brain is efficient and values getting things done.[9]

Clearly, Process is a right-hemisphere kind of state. Process is not about accomplishing anything. You do Process just to do it, and it's not even really about doing; it's about being in the unending present moment. Process is about setting aside details, demands, and judgments and allowing yourself to forget about boundaries and time constraints.

Taylor observes, "My right mind is open to new possibilities and thinks out of the box. It is not limited by the rules and regulations established by my left mind that created the box. Consequently, my right mind is highly creative in its willingness to try something new. It appreciates that chaos is the first step in the creative process."[10]

The true value of Process is that it gives us fifteen to thirty minutes to be free of the demands of the usually dominant left hemisphere to mess around with small-scale chaos to find the creative gifts of the right hemisphere.

WRITER'S APPLICATION: WHEN IS WASTING TIME NOT A WASTE OF TIME?

Make no mistake: The left hemisphere is just as important as the right in achieving our writing dreams. People who indulge in right-brain dreaming without harnessing the power of the left brain to get things done spend their entire lives waiting for a someday that never arrives. However, devoting fifteen to thirty minutes a day to let the right hemisphere take the lead during Process is not going to damage our ability to accomplish our goals, however much the left hemisphere may protest about wasting time. Significantly, Taylor observes, "the last thing a really dominating left hemisphere wants is to share its limited cranial space with an open-minded right counterpart!"[11]

I can always see the wheels turning in people's minds when I suggest Process. I know their left hemisphere is thinking something along the lines of, "That sounds silly. Childish, even. How can I justify taking time to just fool around when I'm not even going to have some result to show for it?" The idea of playing just to play is too decadent to accept at first.

As I explain the value of Process, most students and clients get an intellectual understanding and are willing to trust me enough to try it. But even the most willing find they are surprisingly resistant to actually doing Process on a regular basis. The inner critic gleefully and viciously attacks attempts to have fun and play around with creativity, saying things like, "This is silly. What a waste of time! You'll never get this. Go do something worthwhile! This is getting me nowhere."

The most insidious self-sabotage says something like, "Sure, I'll do Process, but not right now. Right now I have these other pressing things to take care of." There will always be pressing priorities. If you postpone Process because of that, there will never be time for it. Without Process, the wellspring of your creative energy and inspiration will run dry. Your Product Time writing, the writing you care deeply about, will go flat and stale, and your inner critic will be the only one who's happy.

But those who persist in building a Process habit report that it is an amazing source of creative energy and insight. YA novelist Betsy H., who was among the most resistant to the idea of Process, startled herself with the realization that she genuinely missed her Process habit when her old practice had to shift to accommodate a new work schedule.

"I never thought I'd say this," Betsy told me, "but I need to find a new Process activity. I'm noticing that I'm not as free in my Product Time without doing Process."

Practicing Process is an antidote to perfectionism. It's a great relief for perfectionists to realize that the old motto, "Anything worth doing is worth doing well"—that is, perfectly—doesn't always apply. Process opens our awareness to the truth that anything worth doing . . . is worth doing.

Pianist and writer Katie H. found that Process gave her a new freedom. "I am often so worried about the final product that I have trouble getting started. I want to know exactly where I am going before I take the first step so I don't waste any time wandering about. Creative Process is a great way for me to steer my attention toward the doing rather than the being done. One of my favorite creative processes is dancing, since it exists entirely in the doing. When I turn music on in my living room and allow my body to move freely, I have no concern for whether one movement leads logically to the next one or whether the movements together form a cohesive whole. When I am done, there is no end product to observe or critique."

Ultimately, the willingness to "waste time" fooling around with Process is what gives us the creative energy, insight, openness, freedom and willingness to make Product Time—the writing that "really counts"—pay off.

When and How

I recommend you give yourself fifteen to thirty minutes a day, five or six days a week to play with Process. You can do the same thing every day, or you might select three or four activities to choose from on any given day. You need a short list of options so you don't spend more time figuring out what to do for Process than actually doing it. Make sure you have whatever materials you'll need on hand; it's frustrating at best and self-sabotage at worst to not have the Play-Doh or scrapbooking supplies you need on the day you decide to make that your creative play.

If you find you spontaneously want to do something unplanned for Process on any given day, and you have the supplies you need, go for it. If you don't have the supplies, get them after doing something else for Process so you'll have them on hand for another day.

Wandering a craft or stationery store shopping for supplies can be Process, but if your house is full of art or writing supplies already, shopping is probably a resistance tool for you and therefore not a good Process choice. Consider shopping an errand and reserve your Process time for the actual play.

I find it's easier to build and sustain a Process habit when you make time for it first thing in the morning. Our brain waves are significantly different when we first wake up; we have more alpha, theta, and delta waves and fewer beta waves. Beta waves are the fastest brain waves (above twelve cycles per second) and associated with logical, concrete thinking and active, waking attention, so we experience fewer of these brain waves when we first wake up. Alpha waves are the second-fastest (between nine and eleven cycles per second) and associated with resting, daydreaming, detached awareness, and a receptive mind; theta waves are third (between four and eight cycles per second) and associated with light sleep and intuition and inspiration; finally, delta waves are the slowest (less than four cycles per second) and associated with deep sleep and deep meditation. Alpha waves seem to be a bridge between conscious and unconscious; the content of dreams and meditation (dominated by theta and delta waves) can be recalled only if you also had alpha waves during the experience.[12, 13]

According to Anna Wise, author of *The High-Performance Mind*, optimum cognitive performance (including greater creativity) occurs when these four brain waves are present and balanced (that is, no one wave is dominant).[14] So we're closer to the creative flow state, where all four brain waves are present and balanced, in the morning than we will be for the rest of the day, when our high-speed beta waves will dominate. This makes mornings a prime time to write or to do Process. Besides, once you start your "regular day," it's too easy to get caught up in the crisis du jour and forget the habits that give you what you need to get through the day.

But if mornings are already jam-packed for you and you're already getting up as early as you're willing to, then mornings are simply not your best Process time. Take a look at your schedule and decide when you can do Process: during your lunch hour, afternoon break or evenings? Because Process will slow your brain waves, it can be a relaxing way to settle your energy before bed. Some research suggests that evenings may be particularly good Process time for extroverts (introverts seem to be more creative in the morning).[15]

If you want help slowing your brain, you can listen to relaxing music while you do it (unless your Process is fooling around with an instrument and you don't want the distraction). But no, it's generally not a good idea to do Process while watching TV. Multitasking is antithetical to Process.

CHALLENGE: START A PROCESS HABIT

I suggest you copy and fill out the Process Commitment Form below. (You can copy the PDF of this form at http://BaneOf YourResistance.com/around-the-writers-block-forms/.) Sign and date it. Ask a friend to sign and date the form as your witness to make the commitment real. Post the completed, signed and dated form in your planner or calendar, on your mirror or in your work-space. Reserve the time in your calendar or planner for your Process commitments.

**My Process choices are (fill in as many or few options
as you like):**

1. _____

2. _____

3. _____

4. _____

I will do Process for (number of) _____ minutes a day
on (number of) _____ days of the week
on (list the days) _____

_____

in the (indicate morning, afternoon or evening)

_____.

Signed: _____ Date: _____
Witnessed by: _____ Date: _____

The more detailed you are in making your commitment to Process, the more likely you are to do it. Having specified days and a regular time for Process significantly helps in making Process a sustainable habit that supports your writing. But be flexible enough to accommodate the unexpected. If you commit to doing

Process five days a week, Monday through Friday, and you miss Tuesday, you can count Monday, Wednesday, Thursday, Friday and Sunday as your five days. You've honored your commitment. Likewise, if you don't get to do your Process at the time you commit to, you can do it earlier or later in the day and it still counts. But if you don't do your fifteen minutes on Tuesday, doing Process for thirty minutes on Wednesday doesn't "make up" for missing Tuesday. You still need to add Saturday or Sunday to honor the commitment to five days.

Start with small commitments you know you can honor. Three or four days a week for ten or fifteen minutes a day is a good place to start; later you can build on your success to expand to five or six days. It's better to say you'll do less and succeed than to overcommit and fail. Showing up for Process for three days for fifteen minutes is a success if you committed to three days for fifteen minutes, but it's a disappointment if you committed to four days for fifteen minutes or to three days for twenty-five minutes. Small commitments regularly honored will build momentum and rebuild your trust in yourself. They also develop and strengthen those neural pathways we talked about at the end of chapter one.

Taking your commitment to Process seriously—by making time to play for the sake of play, refreshing your creative spirit and restoring your creative energy, surrendering your expectations and demands, abstaining from slavish devotion to constant productivity and unending agendas, and being willing to experiment and explore the new creative territory—fortifies your ability to resolve the resistance that has kept you from the writing you want and need to do. But most important, keep your Process time fun and light! This is play, after all. We use the word "commitment" to impress other people who might want to take your time. "Sorry, I can't do it; I have another commitment" sounds more official and unassailable than, "Sorry, I'm playing."

INQUIRY

"What would be fun to play with? What did I love to fool around with when I was a kid that might be fun to revisit? Have I lost track of the value of play, and if so, how do I regain it?"

HABIT TWO: PRODUCT TIME

Success Story

Screenwriter and novelist Miriam Queensen observes, "Giving myself permission to write, even for just a short time, and not waiting for 'perfect conditions' for writing provided me with just the impetus I needed to get moving. I'd been stuck for quite a while, not even sure which project to work on first. So I was paralyzed and didn't write at all."

When she committed to Product Time along with Process and Self-care, Miriam started writing every day she planned to write. "I started out with only ten to fifteen minutes, but I have learned that I can write one page in fifteen minutes. Just the fact that I write a little every day keeps the novel in my mind, so that by the next day I sit down to write, the next page or more is already there in my head, ready to be typed out, whether I've consciously thought about it or not."

Showing up for Product Time ten to fifteen minutes a day moved Miriam from being stuck on page 50 to completing her novel.

When Is It Process Time; When Is It Product Time?

As I mentioned in chapter three, when you're freewriting, doing morning pages or journaling just to fill the page with no particular outcome in mind, that's what I call Process. If you're freewriting to develop a character, idea or image for a specific piece of writing that you eventually want to share (by publishing, posting on your blog, submitting for a grade or credit, or printing for yourself, friends and family), that writing is Product Time.

When you're searching for your next writing project, it's trickier to tell the difference between Process writing and Product Time writing. If you're playing around just to play, it's probably Process; if you're playing around with an idea or in search of an idea, it's probably Product Time.

The difference lies in your intention. Process is creative play for the sake of play with no expectations about the outcome. It's the in-the-present-moment process of doing Process that matters, not the final results. When you show up for Product Time, on the other hand, you do have an intention that you will create a writing product (hence the term "Product Time"). If what you're doing needs to be done to complete a writing project, that's Product Time.

You need to put in many days of Product Time to do all the work necessary to create a piece of writing you want to share/publish/post/submit/distribute, so not every day's effort will yield the end product you're looking for, but every day's effort contributes to that final product.

Why "Product Time" Instead of "Writing Time"

I use the term "Product Time" rather than "writing time" because "writing time" implies drafting, revising, editing and proofing. Product Time is that, of course, but it's much more. Thinking about "writing time" as the time you spend drafting and rewriting is like thinking that making wine is putting wine in a bottle, corking it and slapping a label on the bottle.

Of course, writing is about getting words on the page, but it isn't only about words on the page, just as making wine isn't only about getting wine in the bottles. Product Time is the time you invest in doing any of the many tasks necessary to produce a piece of writing.

WHAT COUNTS AS PRODUCT TIME

Writer Jacquelyn B. Fletcher acknowledges, "The biggest struggle I've had with Product Time is remembering what counts. Because I have a merciless inner critic who berates me for laziness, I have to remind myself again and again that research counts!

Interviews count! And the writing, too. Showing up at the desk for Product Time moved me from dreams of a writing career to the reality of a writing career."

If a task needs to be completed to finish a writing project, the time you spend doing that task should be considered Product Time. Product Time will include:

- Finding an idea
- Researching (both research that's focused on a specific topic and exploratory research that's part of finding your next writing idea or project), including reading, Internet searches, interviews, questionnaires, surveys, field research, etc.
- "Incubating" the idea
- Freewriting
- Clustering (a.k.a. bubble brainstorming), mind-mapping, creating a fishbone diagram, or using any other brainstorming technique
- Making lists
- Writing character sketches or the backstory
- Storyboarding or outlining
- Describing, drawing or mapping the setting
- Researching potential publishers/publications, including reading and analyzing sample issues or previously published books, reviewing writer's guidelines
- Writing and submitting query letters or cover letters
- Drafting
- Editing, revising and rewriting
- Proofing

- Enlisting readers and requesting feedback
- Providing feedback to members of a writer's group
- Doing exercises or responding to writing prompts
- Taking a writing class
- Writing a synopsis or book proposal

If you sit down with the intention to do your Product Time and you don't do anything else—don't distract yourself with email, Twitter, Facebook, blog stats, voice mail, TV, texting, Internet shopping, looking for answers in the refrigerator, or sorting your junk drawer—you're doing Product Time. Even if you end up staring at the spot where the ceiling meets the wall, pondering and puzzling over what the heck you're going to do with this piece, as long as you show up and make yourself available to your writing, that counts as Product Time. This is a valuable investment. Give yourself credit for it.

Don't worry—your capacity to sit for ten or fifteen minutes day after day truly doing nothing is much smaller than you might think. If you keep showing up, you'll start doing something that moves your writing forward. The real challenge is to stop distracting yourself and running away.

INSIDE THE WRITER'S BRAIN: TAKING THE SCARY OUT

All of us have a mix of positive and negative responses to our writing. The brain remembers negative experiences differently than positive ones. When you experience something dangerous or threatening, you tend to remember lots of incidental details so your limbic system can react to them in the future (because anything associated with the previous danger could be part of the danger, and from a survival perspective, it's better to overreact to something that's benign than to not react to something that's dangerous).

As you may recall from Aimee's story in chapter two, your limbic system will respond even if you don't remember the previous negative experience. This is the origin of the unsettled, anxious feeling so many writers get when we sit down to write or think about writing. Our brains have learned that writing can be scary.

Fortunately, the nature of neuroplasticity means we can retrain our brains. With a lot of repetition of positive experiences, we can learn that showing up to write doesn't have to be scary. We'll review when and how to reward yourself in chapter seven; for now, know that giving yourself a small treat every time you show up for Product Time and letting yourself feel good about your accomplishment is part of retraining your brain that writing is not dangerous.

Dr. Mary Maloney, a professor in the Management Department at the University of St. Thomas, learned to stop seeing writing as a threat. Mary writes not because she has a secret passion to write the great American novel or publish her memoirs—she writes because she has to. "I've never enjoyed writing, but it's a necessary part of my job. I'd put off writing up my research, then kill myself meeting a deadline, then dislike writing even more based on that unpleasant experience, then go on to procrastinate my next project."

Mary's fear and desperation made it much more difficult for her to write than it had to be, and made her writing less effective than it could be.

After we talked about the neurology of resistance and how her anxiety and resistance put her limbic brain in charge and silenced her cortex, Mary learned new habits to retrain her brain. Instead of waiting until she absolutely had to start writing a paper or manuscript, she challenged herself to put in fifteen minutes of Product Time a day, five days a week (along with practicing Process and Self-care). As Mary built her Product Time habit, she realized that she actually enjoyed some writing-related tasks, like documenting the results of her research. Expanding her idea about what counts for Product Time allowed her to start "writing" sooner, refine her analysis, improve the final product, and more fully appreciate the aspects of research that she is passionate about. While writing journal articles will never be Mary's passion, it's no longer scary.

Showing Up Is Key

Showing up isn't half the battle; it *is* the battle.

Spike Carlsen, author of *A Splintered History of Wood* and *Ridiculously Simple Furniture Projects*, believes writers—and our writing—yearn for the structure that showing up for Product Time gives us. "When I was raising five mutinous teenagers, people would often expound, 'They may act like they don't like structure and discipline—but deep down inside, they yearn for it.' So it is with writing: Your words may play hooky, sulk, roll their eyes at you, hang out with the wrong prepositional phrases, but deep down inside, they like Product Time. It provides them with structure—and the subliminal peace of mind that comes with it. Someday your words will thank you for it."

For some writers, the idea of "Product" Time can sound in-timidating. Emerging novelist Dr. John Drozdal observes, "Before I really understood what Product Time meant, I was under the impression that I had to 'produce something' and I wasn't sure I could handle the pressure. Once I understood that the commitment is to show up to write, I discovered that it actually reduced the anxiety. Now I look forward to that time. And I'm writing."

Keeping the promise to show up is essential. Norman Mailer points out in *The Spooky Art: Some Thoughts on Writing*, "If you tell yourself you are going to be at your desk tomorrow, you are by that declaration asking your unconscious to prepare the material. . . . You have to maintain trustworthy relations. If you wake up in the morning with a hangover and cannot get to literary work, your unconscious, after a few such failures to appear, will withdraw."[1]

Mailer observes that you can recover trust with your unconscious—the source of all your imagination and innovation—but you have to earn it. You earn it by showing up even if you think you have nothing to write, even if you feel restless or think there's something else "more important" that you should be doing. Showing up every time you say you will, no matter what else is going on that day, builds and maintains the neural pathways for writing (a.k.a. your writing habit).

When you show your unconscious you are sincere and trustworthy, you will find your unconscious is generous in its forgiveness. Your mind will sparkle with exciting images and intriguing ideas and you'll have plenty to work with in your Product Time.

How to Evaluate Product Time

NaNoWriMo (National Novel Writing Month) participants and some well-known authors like Stephen King keep track of their writing in terms of how many words they string together—50,000 words in the month of November for NaNoWriMo, 2,000 words a day, 365 days a year for Mr. King. Keeping track of word counts can be very effective when we are drafting and generating new material.

The problem with relying exclusively on word counts to evaluate your Product Time is that, as we'll see in the Stages of the Creative Process table, there are six stages in the creative process, and in only one of those six stages do we actually have pen on the page or fingers on the keyboard generating words to count. If we think word counts are the only measure of how hard we're working and how much progress we're making, we will be very discouraged while we're in any of the other five stages. Because word counts cannot account for all the work we do throughout the entire creative process, overreliance on them can demoralize us and generate the very anxiety and resistance we need to avoid.

This is why I tell my students and coaching clients to keep word counts if they wish while they're drafting, but they will be best served by evaluating their Product Time throughout all stages of the creative process not by how many words or pages they write or how good the writing is, but simply by whether or not they show up.

Stage	Characteristics	What to Do in This Stage
FIRST INSIGHT	The first glimpse of the idea. See the whole (the big picture) and the holes in it. Recognize that what's missing or problematic is a creative opportunity.	Ask open-ended questions. Maintain or pretend ignorance. Freewrite. Cluster. Brainstorm. Mind-map.
SATURATION	Immerse yourself in information. Seek facts, data, details from a variety of sources. Information leads to more questions and the search for more information.	Research and analyze audience. Clarify the purpose. Research via reading, interviews, questionnaires, surveys, field research, etc. Record research results and cite sources as you go.

INCUBATION	The conscious mind is unable to process all the information gathered in Saturation and begins to falter. Frustration or anxiety can result. The conscious mind must surrender so that the unconscious mind can work on the problem to create new associations and connections.	Procrastinate. Nap. Walk. Leave the work to do something else. Get your body busy. Freewrite. Ask yourself questions and freewrite answers. Cluster. Brainstorm. Talk to others. Explain it to someone else.
ILLUMINATION 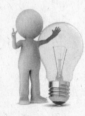	Everyone's favorite stage. The flash of insight. The "aha" or "eureka" moment when it all fits together, when the conscious mind has awareness of the solution presented by the unconscious.	Freewrite. Cluster . Mind-map. Make lists. Brainstorm. Don't talk to others here.
VERIFICATION 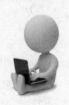	Making the Illumination tangible by writing the piece, painting the painting, etc. You make the creative insight and solution something that can be shared with others.	Write draft. Do *not* try to draft, edit and proof at the same time. Revise, edit, rewrite. Cut and paste. Talk to others (but do limit this). Ask for feedback. Read out loud. Proofread.

HIBERNATION 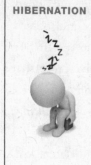	Often Verification leads back to First Insight, and the cycle is repeated to perfect the creative product. Sometimes the completion of a creative project takes so much creative energy, we're drained. Nothing new can develop in this fallow time. The reserves must be refreshed.	Let the writing sit. Wait. Do something that recharges your energy and refreshes your creative spirit. Look at beautiful images or get yourself outside. Work on another project. Talk with others. Proofread.

Stages of the Creative Process

The Stages of the Creative Process table identifies the characteristics of the six stages in the creative process and what kinds of work a writer can do in each stage. Notice that although you may be freewriting or recording questions and answers in a journal during several stages, only in Verification do you draft, edit and revise. What most people think of as "writing time" occurs in the Verification stage. You can't get to Verification without working your way through the previous four stages. You need to give yourself time and credit for all your creative work.

In *Dancing in the Dragon's Den: Rekindling the Creative Fire in Your Shadow*, I referenced the five-stage creative process Betty

Edwards describes in *Drawing on the Artist Within* and added a sixth stage, Hibernation, based on my experience and observations as a teacher and coach. (For more details on the first five stages and the evolution of ideas about the creative process, see *Drawing on the Artist Within*;[2] for more information on Hibernation and the significance of the stages to resistance, see *Dancing in the Dragon's Den*.)[3]

Edwards suggests that different stages require different kinds of thinking, what she calls L-mode and R-mode (referring the left and right hemispheres). These correspond to Dr. Jill Bolte Taylor's description of hemispheric differences reviewed in chapter three. L-mode is a style of thinking that relies on the logical, linear perceptions and interpretations the left hemisphere excels in, and R-mode is a style of thinking that relies on the fluid, circular perceptions and interpretations of the right hemisphere. According to Edwards, First Insight, Incubation, and Illumination are mainly R-mode, while Saturation and Verification are mainly L-mode. I disagree with Edwards only in the case of Illumination, which I'm convinced is equally R- and L-modes.

Since the styles of thinking and the function of each stage are different, the kinds of activities a writer needs to do to move through each stage also vary. What you'll do in Product Time varies depending on what stage you're in. Don't worry if you're not sure what stage you're in—as long as you show up and do something related to your writing, you've honored your commitment to Product Time.

First Insight

This is the preliminary stage of discovering what you want to write about or what problem you want to solve. It is that first glimmer of an idea you get when you see the whole picture and recognize what's problematic or missing (the holes within the whole, in other words) as creative possibilities. Many writers in First Insight feel guilty about wandering aimlessly in search of something to write about, not realizing this is what First Insight is all about. It's vital in First Insight to ask lots of open-ended, "what if?" "why not?" "how about?" questions. Assuming you know the answers prevents you from recognizing the possibilities inherent in First Insight.

During First Insight, it's not so much what you do in Product Time as how you do it. This is when reading News of the Weird, watching seemingly random video clips and documentaries, or reading whatever happens to strike your fancy will intersect with your life experiences to give you a flicker of inspiration.

Activities that open your mind without focusing it too much are good for First Insight. Power walking won't move you through First Insight, but aimless wandering walks in museums, galleries, quirky shops, and beautiful natural places will. Give yourself permission to flip through and read bits and pieces of whatever books and magazines fall your way in libraries, bookstores and waiting rooms and from friends. Open a writing book to a random page and try the first writing exercise or prompt you find.

Product Time during First Insight can include watching TV and videos, as long as you avoid the stuff that makes your mind numb, focusing instead on stuff that makes you say, "Really? I never thought about that." For me, programs on PBS, Discovery, the Science Channel, the History Channel and Bravo are good fodder. For you, it might be a different combo. You'll do a lot of freewriting, journaling, clustering, and mind-mapping. If you're not sure where to start when you're in First Insight, use the Interest Inventory below.

Interest Inventory

If you know you want to write, but don't know what you want to write, list five of each of the following:

- hobbies, interests or things you like to do or have always wanted to try
- things you're passionate about
- qualities or traits you value in yourself and others (e.g., honesty, courage, generosity)
- issues or situations that outrage you
- questions you've always wondered about
- people you admire (living or dead or fictional)
- magazines, other publications and types/topics of books you read
- groups, associations, clubs or loose affiliations you're a member of
- things or people that caught your attention or interested you today
- topics you might want to write about someday

- groups or types of people who might be interested in these topics (Note: Some writers find that thinking about who else might be interested in a topic helps them clarify what and how they want to write. Some writers find that thinking about potential audiences too soon is overwhelming or too limiting. If thinking about audience inhibits you, skip this one.)

Use your Product Time every day to freewrite about one of the things in any of the lists on this Interest Inventory. When you realize you want to find out more about a topic, use your Product Time to explore the topic (i.e., do some research). If your interest in the topic wears out, come back to this Interest Inventory. If your interest remains, congratulations—you've found a writing project.

Saturation

In the second stage, you immerse yourself in data, details and facts. This is when you start looking for answers to some of the open-ended questions you asked in First Insight. You want to get as much information as you can from a variety of sources. This includes research on the subject matter you're writing about or research to clarify what you want to write about next. It's also research you do on the publishing end—investigating agents, publishers and publications.

Do anything that brings in data during your Product Time in Saturation. Read everything that could be relevant: books, academic journals, diaries, journals, notes, magazines, correspondence. The Internet makes getting information easier than it's ever been;

your challenge is to sort through the information (and misinformation) the Internet can bury you in. You can interview people: in person, on the phone, via email or online chats. You can also observe people—watch how they move and interact, listen to how they talk and what they don't say. You can conduct your own field research, questionnaires, surveys, focus groups, etc., or read through the findings of other researchers. If you're writing memoir, you can flip through family photo albums, diaries, journals and other documents to trigger memories and associations. It's helpful to list the questions you want to answer and to use a system to keep track of what you find and where.

Incubation

When all the research you're doing starts to overwhelm you, you enter the Incubation stage. The typically dominant left hemisphere can't keep track of all the data and details, facts and figures you've accumulated. You're eager to move ahead and get to the writing, but you can't quite figure out how it all fits together. Your right hemisphere is working to discover new associations and connections, but you're not consciously aware of this, and it's easy to feel frustrated with a perceived lack of progress. You may wish you could force your way through to produce something, but you can't. If you measure your success only with external measures of production, like words or pages written, you'll feel very discouraged, which is why incubation is often mistaken for writer's block, when it actually is a normal part of the process.

Incubation is about unseen growth. If you open an incubating egg prematurely to check its progress, you kill the chick. Just because you can't see it doesn't mean there isn't something significant happening.

If you think of the creative process as a jigsaw puzzle, Saturation is when you gather all the pieces of the puzzle and lay them out on the table. Incubation is when you realize just how jumbled the pieces (facts) are and begin to wonder whether you'll ever be able to make sense of them. If you expect that you'll instantly see how all the pieces fit together or that the puzzle will magically put itself together as you pour it out of the box, you're going to be very frustrated. Besides, if you could immediately see how the pieces fit together, the puzzle would be so simple it would bore you. To the right hemisphere, moving the pieces around, seeing what fits where, looking for patterns and associations is the fun part.

What you need to do in Product Time during Incubation is not going to look enough like work to satisfy the left hemisphere. This is the one stage where showing up for Product Time could well mean abandoning your usual work space to take a nap, go for a walk, work out or wander away to do something else. You need to find something to keep your left hemisphere busy enough to butt out and let your right hemisphere do the real work of this stage. During Incubation it can be very effective to combine Process and Product Time—give your hands something to manipulate (clay, colors, paper) and your left hemisphere will stop chattering and distracting your right hemisphere's search for meaning. You can ask yourself questions and freewrite possible answers (but don't expect the answers to make complete sense yet). You can cluster, brainstorm, talk to others, and try to explain what you know so far. Like First Insight, it's not so much what you do in Incubation as how you do it: give yourself permission to not know, to aimlessly move the puzzle pieces around, and, most of all, to find ways to stay in motion while you wait.

Illumination

Eventually, your stumbling around in Incubation will lead you to the glory of Illumination. Illumination is everyone's favorite stage. It's the flash of insight when you can see how it works, the eureka moment when all the pieces fit together. It tends to be a brief flash, perhaps because it requires both left- and right-hemisphere perception and most of us are accustomed to using one or the other, not both together. Because Illumination has such a short duration, there is limited time to do much during Product Time.

Your main task in Product Time during Illumination is to simply pay attention. If you're writing fiction or creative nonfiction, Illumination Product Time can be letting the scene unfold in your imagination and recording a few sentence fragments that capture sensory or emotional highlights of the scene. If you're writing poetry, it's playing with the images, sounds, rhythms in your imagination and recording key words or phrases. If you're writing nonfiction, it's paying attention to how the ideas fit together and taking notes. You might have time to capture the inspiration with a freewrite, cluster or mind map. Talking to others during Illumination is not a good idea because it dissipates the creative energy and can easily distract you so much that the new aha insight slips between your fingers.

Verification

This is where you transform the insight and passion of the Illumination into something tangible that can be shared with others. This is the "fingers on the keyboard, pen on the page" stage when you do the things that most people consider "writing."

Product Time during Verification is pretty much what you expect: drafting, reading your work, revising, editing, reorganizing, asking for and incorporating feedback. Brainstorming tools like clustering and mind-mapping are also effective.

On rare occasions, Illumination is lengthened beyond the typical brief flash to allow you to do Illumination and Verification together. At these times, you start drafting almost as soon as you get the flash of insight about how the pieces fit together. When you're lucky, you enter what Mihaly Csikszentmihalyi calls the "flow" state,[4] that blissful experience of seeing or hearing your characters or narrator with your mind's eye or mind's ear, knowing exactly what to write while your fingers race to keep up with the images and ideas flooding your mind.

More frequently, the Verification and Illumination are separate and distinct, and you need to draft, edit and revise from the memory of your last Illumination. Sometimes wrestling with a draft in Verification (a.k.a. editing) gives new inspiration (a.k.a. re-vision). You might have a string of Illuminations each followed by Verification. But typically, new Illumination comes from the willingness to move through Incubation, and Incubation is fueled by the research done in Saturation. This is why Verification usually raises new questions that bring you back to First Insight, and you cycle through the whole progress again.

But sometimes—if you've completed a big project or if you've skimped on your Process—you leave Verification drained of creative energy. The tired, flat feeling that you're crawling through a desert without an oasis in sight is the sign that you've entered Hibernation.

Hibernation

Like Incubation, Hibernation is sometimes mistaken for a creative block because you simply don't have the energy or insight to do anything creative. And like Incubation, Hibernation is a normal and natural part of the process. Writers who consistently let themselves play with Process typically experience hibernations that are shorter or less intense, but no one can postpone Hibernation indefinitely. Why would you want to? Hibernation is the equivalent of letting a garden go fallow in the winter. It's the quiet time when you recharge your creative energy and refresh your perspective. The urge to be constantly producing something, constantly busy doing "something important" may be as American as apple pie, but it doesn't serve our creativity. Downtime is essential to long-term creative effectiveness.

Product Time during Hibernation might feel self-indulgent because you need to do whatever will feed your creative spirit: rest, nap, have quiet time alone or in the company of people who don't drain your energy, and spend as much time as you can in beauty. Be in nature, visit museums and galleries, read really good books, flip through coffee table books of photography and art, watch great films. Sometimes you can work on another project—it's not uncommon to be in different stages with different projects—and sometimes you have to work on another project, but when your overall creative energy has been drained, you need to make time to do the things that restore your spirit.

The Second Key: Fifteen Magic Minutes

The first key to making Product Time work for you is to show up and give yourself credit for all the work you do each and every time you show up. The second key is to commit to no more than fifteen minutes.

Eileen Peterson has discovered the magic in fifteen minutes. "The thing that amazes me about Product Time is how much I can get done in only fifteen minutes. Incredible revelations come to me about who my characters really are, what their motivations are, and where the story is going—all within a fifteen-minute session. My novel and essays are getting done in fifteen minutes a day, one day at a time."

Some writers worry that they won't be able to really accomplish much in just fifteen minutes. Unfortunately, these are often writers who haven't accomplished anything for weeks, months or longer because they just can't seem to find big blocks of time for writing. In my opinion, a little something regularly repeated adds up to a whole lot more than what would be a lot of something if you ever got around to it but never do.

Besides, I'm not suggesting that you never do more than fifteen minutes. I'm recommending you *commit* to no more than fifteen minutes a day, four to six days a week. If you work beyond that commitment, fabulous! You can even schedule and reserve a target time beyond the fifteen-minute commitment. But the commitment never goes beyond fifteen minutes.

There is magic in the fifteen-minute commitment, and there's brain science behind that magic.

INSIDE THE WRITER'S BRAIN: THE POWER OF FIFTEEN MAGIC MINUTES

Remember how the limbic system will push the creative cortex out of the driver's seat when you feel threatened or stressed? Planning to sit down and write for hours on end is often stressful enough to trigger a limbic system takeover. One of the biggest benefits of habits is that because they are familiar, they tend to soothe the limbic system and keep the creative cortex engaged.

The smaller the time commitment, the smaller the likelihood of a limbic system takeover. You need a time commitment small enough that you can do it no matter what else happens on any given day, and small enough that you can repeat it four to six times a week. For many writers, that's fifteen minutes; for some it's ten minutes; for some it's five minutes. (Technically, I suppose I should call it the "Magic of No More Than Fifteen Minutes," but "Fifteen Magic Minutes" is more memorable.)

Committing to no more than fifteen minutes goes a long way toward eliminating the resistance so many of us feel before we get started. If you do feel a bit of trepidation, you can reassure your-self, "It's just fifteen minutes. I can do fifteen minutes. It's nothing to freak out about." In other words, you calm your limbic system enough to keep your cortex online.

On a practical level, it's usually easier to find time for and always easier to actually show up for five fifteen-minute sessions throughout the week than to find one seventy-five-minute session when you won't procrastinate, postpone and distract yourself or be interrupted and delayed by others.

Showing up five times a week will create a stronger habit sooner than showing up once a week. The power of habit lies with Hebb's Law, which states that "neurons that fire together, wire together."[5] When a group of neurons frequently fire together or in sequence, a layer of fatty white tissue called myelin insulates the neurons in that neural pathway, making the circuit more effective.[6] The more often you give the collection of neurons you use for writing the opportunity to fire together, the more myelin gets wrapped about those neurons, the stronger the network that connects those neurons becomes, and stronger the habit becomes. Conversely, if you don't consistently give your "writing neurons" the opportunity to focus and fire together on your writing, they'll become part of some other neural pathway, that is, some other habit.

First Things First

First you have to build the Product Time habit. For the first couple of months, focus on showing up for Product Time when you say you will and don't concern yourself with what you're working on or how "good" it is. Until your habit is strongly entrenched as part of your life, what you do is far less important than the fact that you honor your commitment.

At first, this just means putting in Product Time at some point on the days you have committed to working; gradually, you'll hold yourself to a more rigorous standard so that you're showing up at an appointed time of day.

When you have a solid habit of showing up for Product Time, that habit will keep you going even when you're in a stage that's challenging for you, when the topic is difficult, or when you're going through some tricky life issues.

Ten Reasons to Keep the Commitment Small

- A Product Time commitment of no more than fifteen minutes is small enough to not intimidate or overwhelm you, so your limbic system is less reactive.
- If you do feel a little anxious, you can talk yourself down: "It's only fifteen minutes—the world will keep spinning, and my family, friends and colleagues will keep breathing."
- It's easier to find smaller bites of time than big chunks of uninterrupted, unscheduled time.
- Short Product Time sessions are more likely to result in actually showing up repeatedly. Repetition strengthens habits,

and habits, in turn, reduce the likelihood of a limbic system takeover.

- Repetition also builds momentum. Your unconscious will continue to work on the writing challenge even after your conscious mind has moved on to other tasks.

- Small commitments lower expectations. Because you're going to work for such a short time, it's okay that what you do today is imperfect and incomplete.

- Because the time you're committed to is small, you break the task into bite-size pieces, which are easier to start and easier to imagine yourself completing.

- If it's for only fifteen minutes, you can justifiably postpone other tasks. You can reverse procrastination—instead of procrastinating the start of your writing, you procrastinate following the distractions that used to keep you from writing.

- You can envision letting go of all the other things competing for your attention and allow yourself to really focus, because it's for only fifteen minutes. This kind of focus, where we get lost in the writing, is one of the biggest joys of writing.

- A small commitment gets you started, and once you get started, it's easy to keep going.

Past Initial Inertia

Fifteen minutes is usually enough to get writers past their "Initial Inertia." (Newton's First Law states that a body at rest tends to stay at rest; likewise, a writer not writing tends to continue not writing.) Initial Inertia is another name for the paralysis that precedes the limbic system's fight-or-flight response. Keeping the commitment small keeps the cortex driving the bus.

Once writers get started with a small, nonthreatening fifteen-minute commitment, they often get into the zone and want to keep writing beyond that fifteen-minute commitment.

Writer and homeopath Pam McAlister has found that "making a commitment to no more than fifteen minutes of Product Time each day encourages me to show up (rather than making me want to put it off). I almost always spend more than fifteen minutes on Product Time, but even if I only spend fifteen minutes, I still get to feel good about having done what I committed to doing."

WRITER'S APPLICATION:
READY, AIM, WRITE!

Like Pam McAlister, many writers who write well beyond fifteen minutes a day acknowledge that if their commitment were larger, they would skip days when they felt "too busy" or "too stressed" to write. Keeping the commitment small keeps them showing up. Once they get started, they want to keep going, so they reserve time to accommodate that.

John Drozdal discovered that "after a few weeks, I often wrote for more than fifteen minutes. I made sure not to schedule anything right after the Product Time period so that I could take advantage of the momentum."

I have a standard commitment to show up for fifteen minutes of Product Time a day, five days a week, Monday through Friday. At the beginning of the week I look at my calendar to see how much more time I can reserve for Product Time and still honor my other commitments to coaching, teaching and speaking. The time beyond my fifteen minutes is my target time. Targets are stretch goals, not commitments. If I get on a roll and want to keep going, I can. If something unexpected comes up and I have to give up some of my target time, it's acceptable. The fifteen minutes are nonnegotiable.

When you've consistently shown up for the Product Time you said you would for several months, you can then start adding targets for longer writing sessions or specific tasks you want to focus on in the Product Time. But the commitment should never increase beyond Fifteen Magic Minutes.

Jacquelyn B. Fletcher has worked hard to get to the point where "my entire workday is my Product Time. And the funny thing is, the more Product Time I do, the more Self-care and Process playtime I build in as well. When I fulfill my Product Time commitment, the feeling of accomplishment is a major reward. That feeling of success propels me into more Product Time, more accomplishments, finished novels, signed contracts . . . the list goes on!"

You can set a target that varies each day, like I do (e.g., thirty minutes on Monday, two hours on Tuesday, five hours on Wednesday, etc.), or you can set a target for the week (a total of six hours this week). You can also set targets for completing specific milestone tasks (e.g., finish first draft of chapter five by August 1).

Just remember that targets are stretch goals, so there's no guilt, anxiety or regret if a target isn't met.

We need wiggle room in the target dates for completing specific tasks because we are creating something we've never created before. Every book, every poem, every essay is different from the ones we've created before. We can make estimates, but because of the novelty of the task, they are rough estimates. We aren't manufacturing widgets on a production line, so we can't expect assembly-line predictability.

Surrender Illusions of Grandeur and Expectations of Perfection

We'd all like to think that when we get inspired, we'll write amazing prose or brilliant poetry, that we'll get into the flow and the writing process will be easy, even blissfully perfect. So the temptation is to wait for the day when you're that inspired, which is a setup for endless procrastination. The danger is that we start to expect that that's what writing should be: amazing, brilliant, easy, perfect. Thinking you have to do it all and do it perfectly is a setup for a limbic system takeover.

When you're committed to writing for only fifteen minutes, you know you can't do everything. You know you can't write perfect prose or poetry in just fifteen minutes, which frees to you to write something imperfect today that you can refine in your fifteen minutes tomorrow.

To write well, you must be willing to write badly. To eventually write something good, first of all you have to write something, and to write something, you have to be willing to surrender your expectations and demands that what you write today must be great.

We can never tell on any given day whether today will be the day we write amazing stuff or the day we do nothing but shovel dreck, writing what Anne Lamott calls "shitty first drafts." That's why Product Time is never evaluated in terms of how "good" the writing is, only by whether or not you show up. Over the long haul, you will write good stuff—you just can't predict or demand when that will happen.

You have to hold an intention that eventually you will achieve a specific writing goal, and at the same time, you have to surrender all expectations about the quality of any day's writing. Fortunately, Process, where you have no expectations or intentions and play just for the sake of playing, prepares you to maintain this tricky balance.

CHALLENGE: I NEED, I WANT

Talk with a writing ally or trusted friend about a time when you moved easily into your writing, the writing went really well, and you were deeply satisfied with the writing experience. Talking will help you remember details you might not otherwise recall.

Then list what you absolutely have to have to write well, what you prefer, and what you can live with or without. Compare your lists to the reality of your current writing space and time, then create an action plan of what you need to change. In some cases, you can change the situation and the environment; in others, you may need to change your assumptions and expectations.

CHALLENGE: START YOUR PRODUCT TIME HABIT

I suggest you copy and fill out the Product Time Commitment Form below. (You can copy the PDF of this form at http://Bane OfYourResistance.com/around-the-writers-block-forms/) Sign and date your Product Time Commitment Form. Ask a friend to sign and date the form as your witness to make the commitment real. Post the completed, signed and dated form in your calendar, planner or work space. Reserve the time in your calendar or planner (whatever system you use to keep track of your appointments and commitments), recording both commitments and targets (if you have them).

The commitment should be no more than fifteen minutes, five or six times a week. Remember it is better to make a small commitment you keep than a grand commitment you can't honor. If you want to reserve time beyond the fifteen-minute commitment so you can keep writing when you're on a roll, you can indicate that in the spaces for your target. Or you can indicate a specific task you want to focus on as your target. Remember the commitment is nonnegotiable—no matter what, you'll do the commitment—and the target is a stretch goal. If you honor your commitments but don't meet all your targets, you still celebrate your success with no guilt or regrets.

My Product Time choices are: (list a single, specific writing project or multiple projects or "discovering my next writing project"; you may not need all four lines)

1. _____

2. _____

3. _____

4. _____

I will show up Product Time for (number of) _____ minutes a day (**no more than fifteen minutes**)

on (number of) _____ days of the week

on (list the days) _____

_____

in the (indicate morning, afternoon or evening)

_____ .

My targets are: (list number of minutes a day or total number of minutes for the week or a milestone you want to reach, such as "draft chapter four" or "revise query letter"; you can list different targets for each day or have just one target for the week or have no target at all)

Monday: _____

Tuesday: _____

Wednesday: _____

Thursday: _____

Friday: _____

Saturday: _____

Sunday: _____

Signed: _____ Date: _____

Witnessed by: _____ Date: _____

INQUIRY

"If I could write anything at all, and I knew it would be successful, what would I write?"

5

HABIT THREE: SELF-CARE

Success Story: You Can't Truly Care for Others If You're Not Caring for Yourself

As a retired RN making writing her second career, Pauline Peterson, author of *Horses for Pauline* and a columnist for *Horse'n Around* magazine, was in the habit of taking care of others. Her patients, family, friends, even her horse had always received more time and attention than Pauline herself. She says it was in the Writing Habit class, where Self-care is recommended, expected and applauded, that she "recognized what I needed and what I could do for myself. It was the power of Self-care that got me unstuck and working regularly on my next book."

Pauline also sees how taking care of herself is a gift she shares with others. "As I took better care of myself, it gave others around me permission to do the same. If I start to get short-tempered with my family, I realize it's because I haven't done enough Self-care, and I know what to do about that before it interferes with my writing or harms my relationships."

Self-care

Pauline's experience and the Inside the Writer's Brain sections in this chapter illustrate that Self-care is not selfish indulgence; it is vital to us as writers and as human beings. Major airlines recognize the basic logic of Self-care when they remind passengers to be sure their own oxygen mask is in place before attempting to assist others. If you pass out because you didn't take care of yourself, you are no good to anyone else.

It can feel selfish to make time for yourself, but it's not. Time for yourself and time for others are opposite, but interdependent, ends of one continuum. We need to do both—getting stuck on one end serves no one. If you make time for only yourself, you are selfish. You'll also be isolated, lonely, stale, uncreative and restless. But if you make time only for others, you're a selfless doormat, unable to create significant work. If you lose sight of who you are, not only will you be unhappy, you can't truly be of service to anyone. The completely selfless also end up feeling isolated, lonely, stale, as well as unappreciated.

Your creative genius is the goose that lays the golden eggs. If you, like the shortsighted farmer in the fable, don't care for the goose, you'll never see another golden egg and neither will anyone else in your community. You need both time for yourself and time with others.

Self-care is anything you do to care for yourself and to maintain your ability to write. If you're already going to the gym to work out because you want to be physically fit, that's a form of Self-care. Simply add the awareness that your workout keeps you creatively fit as well.

There are many ways to care for yourself. This chapter will explore five major forms that are most beneficial to writers: adequate sleep, exercise, meditation, time to focus, and play. You don't have to take on all five at once; start with making a habit out of one kind of Self-care. When that practice is firmly entrenched as part of your routine, you can focus on creating a habit out of another form of Self-care. After all, it's not really caring for yourself if you work out regularly but never get enough sleep, for example. Self-care means caring for your whole self. Eventually, you'll want to give yourself time for most, if not all, the major forms of Self-care.

Success Story: Self-care, Not Self-indulgence

Copywriter and novelist Laura Sommers learned to distinguish real Self-care from self-indulgence that's disguised as Self-care. "Self-indulgence might look like Self-care on the surface," she acknowledges, "but instead of giving me that deep sense of satisfaction that Self-care brings, it leaves me feeling flat."

Taking a nap, taking a break or treating yourself can be legitimate Self-care at times, but Laura observes that those kinds of things can slide into self-indulgence if she's not paying attention. "Self-indulgence is taking a nap I don't need instead of reading a book. Or staring at the TV for hours, thinking of numerous things I could be doing—things I always say I wish I had time to do, but now don't seem willing to leave the couch to do. It's feeling sorry for myself and thinking I deserve a break because I'm busy. It's rewarding myself with junk food or dessert or wine one time too many. It's going for the 'quick hit' stimuli, like shopping or re-arranging furniture or writing clever emails."

When Laura finds herself overindulging, she asks herself why. "Usually it means it's time to drop something unimportant to make time for something that matters, but that scares me a little."

True Self-care gives Laura what she needs to be the writer and artist she strives to be. "Self-care is when I truly take care of my *best* self. And sometimes that means I have to face my fears or create conflicts or make decisions others will question. It's when I make the effort to go to the art show across town, or invite a friend to a concert because my husband hates classical music. It's when I turn down a social opportunity on a busy day because I really need to run two miles, and I know I can only do one or the other. Or it's calling a friend for lunch because she always makes me feel good about my creativity. It's not just taking care of my dear self in a superficial way—that's the path that puts me on the couch staring at the TV. It's knowing my true self, and doing what my true self needs to thrive."

INSIDE THE WRITER'S BRAIN: THE POWER OF DOING NOTHING

Studies show that when rats experience something new, their brains create new patterns of activity. But to create a long-term memory—in other words, to really learn from the experience—the rats must take a break. Apparently learning, for both rats and humans, happens not so much in the moment of the experience as in the rehearsing and reinforcing of the new neural patterns that occur after the experience.

The *New York Times* quoted Dr. Loren Frank, assistant professor of physiology at the University of California, who specializes in learning and memory, as saying, "Almost certainly, downtime lets the brain go over experiences it's had, solidify them and turn them into permanent long-term memories." Frank believes that when you constantly stimulate your brain, "you prevent this learning process."[1]

This much-needed downtime is a bonus you'll gain in addition to the unique benefits found in each of the five types of Self-care we'll discuss in this chapter.

ADEQUATE SLEEP

Success Story: Perchance to Achieve a Dream

Lisa B., an accomplished children's author with more than forty books to her credit, wanted desperately to write a YA novel. And desperate was how she felt about it—until a routine doctor's appointment revealed that she had sleep apnea. Within a month of getting her sleep machine and hence the sleep she needed, Lisa noticed the change in her writing. "The block I had around writing fiction for older kids just melted away. I know that finally getting the sleep I needed was a huge part of that."

INSIDE THE WRITER'S BRAIN: SLEEP ON IT

A sleep-deprived brain is a creatively impaired brain. Sleep deprivation has devastating consequences for the whole body, and for the brain in particular: memory, mood, alertness and the ability to focus attention, decision making, learning, logical reasoning, creativity and motivation are all impaired. In addition to these cognitive losses, sleep deprivation disrupts hormone balances, depletes the immune system, interferes with metabolism so that the body loses muscle and gains fat, accelerates aging and increases the likelihood of diabetes, heart disease, de-pression, anxiety disorders and serious, even fatal, accidents.[2,3]

In addition to reversing all the physical and cognitive costs of sleep deprivation, getting enough quality sleep improves both the divergent and convergent thinking required for creativity. For all these reasons, sleeping well reduces resistance.

WRITER'S APPLICATION: HOW MUCH IS ENOUGH?

The amount of sleep we need to perform at our best varies widely among individuals and even varies throughout one person's life. Some studies[4] suggest that it's less a matter of how long you sleep than it is a matter of how many sleep cycles you complete. A sleep cycle has five phases: 1) still conscious, but body is relaxed and breathing slowed, primarily alpha waves; 2) light sleep, primarily theta waves; 3) deep sleep, primarily delta waves; 4) REM sleep, dreaming, primarily theta and alpha waves (if alpha waves are absent, dreams won't be recalled); 5) light sleep, primarily theta waves, can be easily awakened by environmental stimuli.

According to Dr. Pierce J. Howard, author of *The Owner's Manual for the Brain*, one of the most important things you can do to improve your sleep is to "organize your time so that you are able to wake up naturally, in a way that does not disrupt a sleep cycle."[5] Use your alarm clock as a backup only; visualize the time you want to wake up and set your alarm for fifteen to thirty minutes later than that.

Some people truly cannot do this, because their job or family situation requires them to wake up at a time that is not natural for them. But before you surrender to the inevitability of unnatural sleep and the toll it will continue to take on your health and well-being as well as your writing, challenge yourself to see how far you can adjust your schedule to accommodate your natural sleep patterns. You will be much more effective during your waking hours.

It's unfortunate that our culture does not respect our need for natural sleep cycles. Many experts agree that sleep deficit is a serious and growing health problem in the United States. The prevailing assumption that the need to sleep is a sign of weakness and that depriving yourself of sleep is a virtue could not be more untrue.

To find out what's natural and effective sleep for you, you might want to start a sleep journal to observe how much you sleep, how many times you woke up during the night (to indicate how many sleep cycles you complete), how you felt when you woke up, and how easily and freely you wrote the next day.

Practice good sleep habits: go to bed at approximately the same time and get the same amount of sleep each night; make sure your bedroom is free of lights and sounds that could interrupt your sleep (even with your eyes closed, ambient light can disrupt your body's clock); don't exercise for several hours before bedtime; have milk or dairy or a light carbohydrate snack before bed; avoid caffeine or artificial sweeteners for several hours before bed; drink alcohol moderately or not at all.

If these suggestions don't help, consult a sleep specialist or go to a sleep lab. Visit the American Sleep Association's website at http://www.sleepassociation.org for more information.

INSIDE THE WRITER'S BRAIN: DREAM MEMORIES, DREAM INVENTIONS

We know we need sleep, but we don't know exactly why or what exactly the brain is doing during sleep. Scans show that the brain is amazingly active while we sleep. In fact, with the exception of the deepest parts of non-REM (nondreaming, phase three) sleep, the brain is more active while we sleep than when we're awake.[6]

Some research suggests that while our body rests in sleep, the brain is busy rehearsing what we learned during the day, improving and solidifying that learning by repeating the patterns we learned during the day hundreds, even thousands of times. The brain does this during REM (dreaming) sleep in short bursts of neural activity at extreme frequencies called sleep spindles. If our sleep is interrupted while a particular pattern is being rehearsed, we do not form a new memory.

Referencing psychology professor James B. Maas, Pierce J. Howard writes, "Without REM sleep and this spindling process, memories dissipate. So if you spend good money learning a new tennis stroke and fail to get a natural night's sleep afterwards, Maas says it is like having never had the lesson. You may remember the elements of the new stroke from an academic perspective, but the absence of spindling fails to convert the motor neural patterns into long-term memory."[7]

Sleep is also when the brain makes new creative associations and connections, as evidenced by so many creative breakthroughs that came to writers, scientists and inventors while dreaming, napping or in a hypnagogic (sleeplike) state. Examples include *Kubla Khan*, *Sophie's Choice*, *Frankenstein*, the periodic table, the structure of the benzene ring, Einstein's theory of relativity, and the sewing machine, among others. Thomas Edison is well-known for napping with ball bearings in his hands; as he relaxed, he would drop the ball bearings, the noise would wake him, and he would record whatever insight he had in that moment.

In terms of brain waves, peak creative experiences are much closer to the brain wave patterns of sleep than those of being awake. Sleep gives us the opportunity to incubate ideas. While our conscious mind is asleep, the unconscious is free to explore new combinations and possibilities. As mentioned in chapter four, napping is an appropriate form of Product Time when you're in the Incubation stage.

EXERCISE

Success Story: On the Move

As a copywriter, novelist, musician, visual artist, gardener, house-holder and business owner, Laura Sommers is usually on the move pursuing personal interests and professional commitments. But she still makes time for exercising a conscious choice.

"I've tried both ways," she says, "and exercising is better than not exercising. When I exercise, I not only feel better in my body and more in the moment, I also avoid the joint stiffness and muscle tightening that make it hard for a writer to sit in a chair for long periods. The most important thing about exercise, by far, is having the ability to start up again when you stop, without judgment or concern that you've 'lost it.' That's the difference between the lifelong exerciser and the binge exerciser. It's also the difference between a writer who writes regularly and someone who writes once or twice a year when inspiration strikes."

Laura continues. "I also have the advantage of a husband who is as passionate about exercising every day as I am about writing. Rather than being jealous of his activity or his physique, I let him be my inspiration to keep at it. I try to see my writing friends the same way. Their activity inspires me to exercise my talent as a writer."

Laura has a variety of exercise options to choose from, including tennis, bicycling, running and walking. "Tennis is great, because when I'm in the middle of a lesson, I'm not thinking about anything else. But after the lesson, I'll see how so much of what I'm learning about tennis relates to learning my craft as a writer, in an oblique sort of way. For example, my instructor teaches the idea that your hand knows how to hit the ball—if you just keep the racquet in the right alignment. From there, it's just practicing keeping the racquet face in the right place as you hit the ball a variety of ways. It's a great message about trusting your instincts, as a tennis player and as a writer. Your writer's hand knows what it wants to do . . . you just have to give it the tools and the practice to do it."

For Laura, exercise burns calories and negative mental states.

"It always restores me. I guess you could say I have faith in the power of exercise to keep me physically and mentally healthy. I don't always feel like taking it on or making time for it, but I *always* feel better after. I sleep better, I breathe better, and I feel more confident about everything, including my writing."

INSIDE THE WRITER'S BRAIN: PUMP UP YOUR BODY, PUMP UP YOUR BRAIN

Exercise doesn't improve just your body; it improves brain function. According to Dr. John J. Ratey, author of *Spark: The Revolutionary New Science of Exercise and the Brain*, the reason it feels so good to move your body is because it helps the brain reach peak efficiency. "In my view, this benefit of physical activity is far more important—and fascinating—than what it does for the body. Building muscles and conditioning the heart and lungs are essentially side effects. I often tell my patients that the point of exercise is to build and condition the brain."[8]

Movement is essential to brain function. Multiple studies have shown that physical exercise improves creativity, memory, reasoning, attention, motivation and problem solving. Ratey cites numerous studies that explain the biochemical reasons exercise has such pervasive, positive effects on the brain. It begins with the fact that physical activity increases blood flow to the brain. The brain is a glutton for glucose and oxygen, using up to 20 percent of the body's energy but representing only 3 percent of the body's overall mass. Both glucose and oxygen are a function of blood flow; the better the blood flow, the better the brain works.[9]

Exercise also increases BDNF (brain-derived neurotrophic factor), what Ratey calls "Miracle-Gro for the brain" because it significantly increases the growth of new neurons and improves their functioning, which in turn improves learning and memory.[10] The presence of BDNF near the synapses also brings in other protein factors—IGF-1, VEGF, and FGF-2—that cause a variety of molecular changes that improve learning and memory.[11]

In addition to increasing the number of neurons, exercise improves the connections between them. Studies at the University of British Columbia show that mice that choose to run on their exercise wheels have significantly more dendrites than mice that don't. More dendrites means more connections between neurons, and the more connected a brain is, the better it functions overall. (Interestingly, mice that are forced to exercise don't show the same improvements as mice that choose to exercise. Fortunately for them, most mice are smarter than humans in this regard and don't have to be forced to exercise.)[12]

Exercise actually stresses the brain and the rest of the body, but without flooding the body with cortisol and other harmful stress hormones. This reverses the negative effects of excessive stress and inoculates you from those negative effects in the future. Stress is like Goldilocks's porridge: too much causes damage, but too little leads to atrophy. Exercise followed by a recovery period provides that "just right" amount of stress that breaks down muscle and neurons slightly and causes them to return even stronger and more resilient after resting.[13]

For many reasons, including the fact that exercise helps regulate the essential neurotransmitters serotonin, dopamine and norepinephrine, exercise improves mood and can be as effective as medication in relieving depression and anxiety disorders.[14,15] In addition to improving mood, higher-than-average dopamine levels are associated with "creativity, the ability to imagine visual scenes in one's head, and the tendency to ask 'what if' questions."[16]

Exercise causes the heart to release ANP (atrial natriuretic peptide), which inhibits the amygdala's role in anxiety and thus calms the brain.[17] People who are physically active are also more likely to be socially active, which in turns has a positive influence on mood.[18]

Since dopamine and norepinephrine are crucial to our ability to focus and pay attention, exercise, especially exercise that includes complex motor skills, improves this cognitive ability as well. (The full significance of this will be highlighted in the upcoming sections on attention.)

WRITER'S APPLICATION: WHAT KIND AND HOW MUCH IS ENOUGH?

Fortunately, you can get the benefits of exercise even if you haven't moved off the couch and out of your office chair for years, and you keep those benefits as long as you keep moving. Individuals vary in their need and desire for exercise, but in general, just about everyone will see positive results from thirty minutes of aerobic exercise two to three times a week. Some benefits (like improving mood and attention) are significantly increased when the frequency is increased to four or five days a week.[19,20]

The gains of aerobic exercise are multiplied when you combine them with activities that require more complex motor skills that challenge and expand synaptic networks.[21] This could include any of the martial arts, figure skating, gymnastics, rock climbing, mountain biking, skateboarding, dance—tango in particular has been noted for positive cognitive and physical effects, in part because the dance is both complex and variable. My personal favorites are geocaching (hiking in different areas using a GPS to find clues and treasure boxes) and dog agility, where the obstacle courses are always different, so that I and my dog get both a mental and a physical workout.

Although an intense workout, defined as 75 to 90 percent of your maximum heart rate (MHR), will significantly increase creative thinking after the workout, it will inhibit learning during the workout.[22] On the other hand, a great deal of anecdotal evidence describes creative breakthroughs occurring while walking, which can be low-intensity (55 to 65 percent of your MHR) or moderate (65 to 75 percent of your MHR), depending on how briskly you walk. So you can probably catch up on your research/reading and even get some interesting new ideas while on the treadmill or elliptical during a moderate or low-intensity workout, but don't plan on retaining much of what you read on the days when you're challenging yourself to hit high-intensity levels.

The brain and body get different benefits from different intensity levels of aerobic exercise; for example, your heart releases ANP only when it's working at moderate or high intensity. To maximize the health and functioning of your brain and the rest of your body, you need to mix moderate and low-intensity activity with occasional high-intensity sprints. Start with the intensity and duration that just challenges your ability to carry on a conversation. As you get more and more fit, you'll need to increase the intensity and/or the length of time to maintain or increase the challenge.

You may also want to vary where you exercise. Some research suggests that exercising outdoors can do more to improve your mood, self-esteem and sense of being rejuvenated and reenergized than the same kind of exercise done inside.[23] Variety in the company you keep during your workouts can also help. Sometimes it's great to be alone with your thoughts, but the "buddy effect" will tend to keep you motivated, and social interaction boosts exercise's ability to promote the growth of new neurons. So consider classes and other ways to be active with others.

Like any of the recommended practices, you'll want to start small and build on your successes. The most important thing is to start moving.

TIME TO FOCUS

Writers at Work—Attention Required

When we put pen to paper or fingers on keyboard to draft or revise, our state of consciousness shifts to a hypnagogic state, a kind of waking, lucid dreaming. We don't lose consciousness of what's happening in the world, but we are so focused on the reality we're creating with words that our awareness of physical reality fades into the background.

"It's a funny state," writes Pulitzer Prize–winning author Robert

Olen Butler in *From Where You Dream*. "It's not as if you're falling asleep at your computer, but neither are you brainstorming. You're *dreamstorming*, inviting the images of moment-to-moment experience through your unconscious. It's very much like an intensive daydream, but a daydream that you are and are not controlling."[24]

John Barth shares Butler's impression of the writer's trance, as do many other writers. In *Writers Dreaming*, Barth says, "Like every writer's professional life, mine is spent doing a kind of dreaming—from the time I sit down at the desk and pick up my faithful fountain pen until the time I put the stuff on the Macintosh—which is a kind of waking up. . . . So much of what we do in those hours when we're actually making sentences, inventing characters and feeling our way through the threads of plot, is hunch and feel—half unconscious and somewhat autohypnotic. Those rituals of getting ready to write seem to conduce a kind of trance state."[25]

Some days we can enter the writer's trance more easily and deeply than others. Easy or difficult, some shift in consciousness is always required to write well. And we can't get there if we are constantly interrupting ourselves with trivia, especially electronic trivia. As writers, we need focus. We are particularly vulnerable to and negatively affected by our culture of distraction.

In *Distracted: The Erosion of Attention and the Coming Dark Age*, Maggie Jackson warns that frequent interruptions decrease creativity and increase stress and frustration. "When you're scattered and diffuse, you're less creative. When your times of reflection are always punctured, it's hard to go deeply into problem-solving, into relating, into thinking. These are the problems of attention in our new world. Gadgets and technologies give us extraordinary opportunities, the potential to connect and to learn. At the same time, we've created a culture, and are making choices, that undermine our powers of attention."[26]

Jackson quotes Arthur Jersild, a developmental psychologist who has researched multitasking. "It is essential for conceptual thought," Jersild says, "that a person give himself time to size up a situation, check the immediate impulse to act, and take in what's there. Listening is part of it, but contemplation and reflection would go deeper."[27]

Writing worth reading must come from the contemplation and reflection of conceptual thought combined with emotional and sensory awareness. As writers we have a responsibility to both think and feel before we blurt. With that responsibility, we must claim our right to have time to think and to sustain our thinking on one topic for more than a few minutes. To restore our splintered attention, we need to refuse to play the distraction game.

INSIDE THE WRITER'S BRAIN: THE MULTITASKING MYTH

If you think doing two or three things at once will save you time, think again. Oh sure, your cerebellum can keep you walking, talking, and chewing gum at the same time, but only because you have practiced these physical activities so much that they are automatic. But when it comes to doing things that require your conscious attention, multitasking is a complete myth and a huge waste of time.

The entire brain system (cortex, limbic system, cerebellum and the rest of the brain stem) may be comparable to a parallel processor. The cerebellum can keep you upright and coordinate the movement of your legs, arms and jaw while your cortex is focused on something else, like which route to take or how to get character A to plot point D.

But the cortex on its own is a sequential processor: it does one task, then shifts attention to do the second task, then shifts attention back to the first, and so on. The cortex can focus on only one thing at a time. Activities that require the cortex's focused attention cannot be done simultaneously.[28]

When you think you're multitasking during your morning commute by driving, putting on your makeup or shaving, changing the radio station, eating breakfast and talking on your cell, you're really shifting your attention from task to task. When you reach for your bagel and remind yourself not to spill cream cheese on yourself, you momentarily lose track of the phone conversation, which means you have to ask the person on the other end of the call to repeat what he or she just said or hope you don't get busted for not paying attention. Meanwhile, your limbic system is about to kick you into panic mode to bring your attention back to the fact that the idiot in front of you has just slammed on the brakes and you just missed your exit.

Every time your cortex shifts attention from one task to another, which it does every couple of seconds, you lose processing speed, accuracy and grace. Trying to multitask takes more time— as much as 50 percent more time in some of the research studies collected by John Medina, author of *Brain Rules*—than to focus on and complete one task before starting another. Add the fact that you're as much as 50 percent more likely to make an error and that some multitasking-induced errors can be serious, even life-threatening, and you start to understand the true cost of the multitasking myth.[29,30]

Not only do attempts to multitask take more time and reduce accuracy, but the more often you try to multitask, the worse it gets. If you are a so-called "frequent multitasker"—that is, you frequently splinter your attention between multiple activities—you're significantly poorer at filtering out irrelevant information, possibly because you're training your brain to try to pay attention to everything. And when tested for their speed of task switching, people who multitask often are slower than those who tend to avoid multitasking.[31]

There are times when multitasking has less severe drawbacks, like when you're multitasking among significantly different activities. The more similar the tasks you're trying to multitask, the more time it takes to shift between them. But different types of tasks, like walking while talking or manipulating clay while reading, require different parts of the brain and don't require the cortex to shift attention between tasks. Thus, these tasks can be done simultaneously with little or no loss of effectiveness in either task.

Different types of tasks don't compete for the same cognitive resources. In fact, they often complement one another, which explains why it helps to give your hands something to do, like play with clay or knit or doodle, when you're struggling to figure out how to word a complex passage.

But for the most part, avoiding multitasking whenever possible is the best strategy. Research shows that the distraction and fractured focus caused by multitasking continues even when you stop multitasking.[32] So multitasking at any time of the day will impair your ability to focus on your writing for the rest of the day.

It is physiologically impossible to give your writing the focused attention it requires while also attempting to check your email, tweet, check your blog stats, and revise a spreadsheet while talking on the phone and keeping one eye on dinner cooking in the next room and what the kids/puppy/cats are up to. Giving yourself time to truly concentrate, especially when you're doing Process or Product Time, is essential.

Preserve Time to Focus

When students tell me they need more discipline, I point out that habits are much more effective than discipline, in part because rigidity and control don't help us ease into the writer's trance. The one place we do need discipline is in maintaining our boundaries. Instead of trying to boss ourselves into being creative, which never really works, we need to put that strict commander part of our personality on guard duty between us and the world, refusing entry to anything that will fracture our focus when we write.

I do Product Time in the morning to protect my ability to focus. Before I check my email or voice mail, before I surf the Internet or read the paper, before I open Excel, QuickBooks, PowerPoint, or any other software program—in other words, before I let the world in—I put in my Product Time. When I have early morning commitments that mean the only way I could do Product Time in the morning would be to get up earlier than is natural for me (and would thus interfere with getting adequate sleep), I do Product Time in the evenings after my partner and I have dinner and relax together. When she goes to bed and the house is quiet, I color or draw for fifteen minutes to settle my mind and then put in my Product Time. I can start Product Time in the middle of the day if I have to, but it's never as effective as starting Product Time first thing. My mind is revved up, I'm trying to remember ten things at once, I'm attending to other people's requests and I simply can't focus on writing projects.

CHALLENGE: WHEN YOU WRITE, WRITE!

For one week, don't do anything but Product Time during your Product Time. Do not multitask. Do not interrupt your Product Time to check your email, shift to another device, program, website or app, look for answers in the fridge, see what your dog/spouse/kids want, or do anything else. Ignore all in-person or electronic bids for your attention for these ten or fifteen minutes. Give yourself the quiet you need to hear your own thoughts and listen to your inner voice.

When you turn on your computer, refrain from using any other electronic device. Don't open any windows other than the file(s) you're working on at that moment. Disable any application that will announce an incoming email, IM or upcoming appointment.

The only exceptions to this rule are:

1. If you're researching, you'll probably use a search engine. But be advised, most Internet research is surface only; to get real depth of information from your source and depth of focus from yourself, you need non-Internet sources. Some studies suggest people comprehend more from reading a hard copy than when they read the same article online. And there's nothing like talking with a real, live person and being able to ask follow-up questions.

2. If you like music in the background, your best bet is instrumentals only. If you're not convinced music with lyrics will interrupt your concentration, try this simple experiment yourself. Try memorizing a list of twenty words while listening to music with lyrics; then test your memory. After a short break, try memorizing a different, but similar, list of twenty words while listening to instrumental music. If you're like most people, you'll see a significant difference in your ability to concentrate.

3. If you write while your infant is down for a nap, do have your baby monitor on. I could suggest that an awful lot of humans throughout history made it through infancy without their parents owning a baby monitor, but I suspect the guilt of turning the monitor off would make it impossible to focus. Anyone who isn't an infant or solely dependent on you for medical reasons should be able to muddle through without you returning a text, call, or email for fifteen minutes.

Even if you live in the Midwest, like I do, and hear a severe-weather siren, there's no need to turn on the radio or TV. Just go to the basement and write there. Believe me, you'll know if a tornado comes through.

It's amazing how much more writing you do when all you do when you write is write.

INSIDE THE WRITER'S BRAIN: THE FUTURE OF FOCUS

Neuroplasticity giveth and neuroplasticity taketh away. The brain's ability to adapt doesn't always serve us. Our nearly constant use of electronics and our cultural expectation that we be constantly and immediately available to everyone and everything through smartphones and cell phones, email, Twitter, Facebook, Google+, other Internet apps, tablet computers, TV, radio, etc. may rewire our brains in ways that make it increasingly difficult to sustain focused attention for more than a few minutes.

A recent article in *The New York Times* provides these statistics:

- In 2008, people processed three times more information each day than they did in 1960.
- People currently spend an average of twelve hours a day exposed to media; in 1960 they spent five hours a day.
- People check email or change windows or computer applications while at work "nearly 37 times an hour." This

means we have an average attention span of just under two minutes!

- Computer users visit an average of forty websites a day, according to research by a supplier of time-management tools.[33]

This same *New York Times* article cites Stanford communications professor Dr. Clifford Nass as saying, "We've got a large and growing group of people who think the slightest hint that something interesting might be going on is like catnip. They can't ignore it. . . . A significant fraction of people's experiences are now fragmented." According to Nass, losing our ability to pay attention is also undermining our capacity for empathy. "The way we become more human is by paying attention to each other."[34] Obviously, empathy is vital to writers; to reach or influence an audience, you have to empathize with them.

CHALLENGE: MAY YOU HAVE YOUR OWN ATTENTION, PLEASE?

Any or all of the following challenges will help you reclaim your own attention.

1. Identify what times of day you are best able to focus your attention. Is it first thing in the morning (like it is for me), or is it midday when you can hole up in the library or coffee shop? Devote some of your most focused time to your Product Time. Perhaps the less obvious step is to allow some of

your most focused time to be downtime; don't wait until you collapse from mental exhaustion.

2. Identify what distracts you and prevents you from focusing on one thing for fifteen minutes. What tempts you to try to multitask? Is it email? IM or text messages? Your phone? People you work with or live with? Your pets? Establish times of the day when you simply refuse to give your attention to these people or things. If you want help, applications like DoNotDisturb and RescueTime will block websites and programs you select for a specified amount of time. Unless you work in an ER or for a bomb squad, no one is going to die and nothing is going to blow up if you don't pay attention to him/her/it for fifteen to thirty minutes. (And if you do work in an ER or for a bomb squad, you know it's vital to give your brain downtime so that when you are working, you can focus completely on the problem in front of you.)

3. Every once in a while, see how much you can get done without your computer and other electronics. At a minimum, Incubation, Illumination, and Hibernation can and should be computer-free. How would you know you're having a eureka moment of Illumination if you're constantly talking or texting on your cell, sending and receiving messages, playing games, and processing information? I've started "email-free Tuesdays and Thursdays" to give myself two days a week when I don't let myself get interrupted by constantly wondering whether I should check my email.

4. List the top ten things or people you worry about. For each, identify one or two specific action steps you can take to alleviate anxiety. Give yourself five or ten minutes a day when you focus exclusively on worry, frustration and fear. Any other time you start to fret, ask yourself what you can do in the moment, and if there is nothing to do, postpone the anxiety until your next "worry session."

5. Create a "time budget." Before attempting to create a monetary budget, experts will tell you that you need to identify how you are currently spending your money. The same is true of time. Before you can intentionally decide how to use your time, you have to know how you are currently spending it. Use the Time of Day Chart on the next page to record how you actually spend your time. If you want to skip the data entry or don't trust yourself to notice how times flies when you're online, check out time-tracking applications like RescueTime. Whether you're recording manually or electronically, gather several weeks of data. Don't judge or feel guilty about how you spend time; this is just information. After you've recorded how you spend time, ask yourself where you want to spend more time. More significantly, consider where you're willing to spend less time so you have time for the things that matter most to you.

TIME OF DAY CHART

	Monday	Tuesday	Wednesday	Thursday	Friday	Saturday	Sunday
12–1 a.m.							
1–2 a.m.							
2–3 a.m.							
3–4 a.m.							
4–5 a.m.							
5–6 a.m.							
6–7 a.m.							
7–8 a.m.							
8–9 a.m.							
9–10 a.m.							
10–11 a.m.							
11–noon							
12–1 p.m.							
1–2 p.m.							
2–3 p.m.							
3–4 p.m.							
4–5 p.m.							
5–6 p.m.							
6–7 p.m.							
7–8 p.m.							
8–9 p.m.							
9–10 p.m.							
10–11 p.m.							
11–midnight							

MEDITATION

Success Story: Quietly, Mindfully Refilling the Well

Freelancer E. S. Fletcher sees a commitment to Self-care as "a reminder that I can't simply draw from my creative well—I also need to replenish it. My favorite way to take care of my creative self is through the silence and stillness of meditation, though I'm not rigid about the method. Most days I meditate—often right before my Product Time—but some days I go for a walk, soak in the tub or I doze with my cats on the couch."

Fletcher applies a variety of Self-care, depending on where she needs the most support on any given day, to nurture what she calls the trinity of mind-body-spirit. "The better my whole self is functioning, the easier it is to get into a creative space because I'm not distracted by that ache in my shoulder or by the errands that need to be run. These practices support me in more than one way: A walk usually clears my head and gives my body the stamina to sit at my desk and write. A catnap slows my body down and relaxes me. Meditation energizes and centers me and helps me transition from the daily dross of life into creative space. It's a simple ritual that helps quiet my chatty, critical left brain and gives my right brain some room to play."

INSIDE THE WRITER'S BRAIN:
DIFFERENT LIFE, DIFFERENT BRAIN

Buddhist monks, lamas, and nuns live a different life from most of us—one of contemplation and service, marked by hours and hours of meditation every day. Because they live a different life, they have different brains. EEG and fMRI brain scans of master meditators (those who have the 10,000–plus hours of practice Malcolm Gladwell correlates to mastery) show increased activity in several areas of the brain, including the insula and caudate (two areas linked to empathy and maternal love), the anterior cingulate, somatosensory cortex, cerebellum and left prefrontal lobe. Meditation decreases activity in the orientation association area in the parietal lobe, which orients you in space and time and allows you to differentiate between yourself and the world.[35] Interestingly, losing the sense of separation between yourself and the world is both a key element in developing empathy and a key characteristic Mihaly Csikszentmihalyi ascribes to the flow state of peak creativity.[36]

Master meditators also show significant increases in gamma waves, while novice meditators show smaller increases. Gamma rays show up when the brain exerts itself, especially when neurons from several areas of the brain are working in concert. "They appear when the brain brings together different sensory features of an object, such as look, feel, sound, and other attributes that lead the brain to its *aha!* moment of yup, that's a lilac bush."[37] Gamma waves seem to be required to achieve the *aha!* of Illumination, the highly prized fourth stage of the creative cycle.

The fact that most of these brain differences are present whether the master meditator is in a meditative state or not means the changes are not just temporary brain states, but consistent brain traits that are the result of structural changes in the brain.[38] The prefrontal cortex and anterior insula, for example, are thicker in the brains of meditators.[39] This implies that writers should be able to draw on the strengths and benefits of meditation not only when we're meditating, but also when we're in the semimeditative state of writing.

As E. S. Fletcher and countless other writers demonstrate, you don't have to be a monk or a nun to bring the benefits of meditation to your writing life. Even novice meditators can see modest improvements fairly quickly. Dr. Richard Davidson, professor of psychology and psychiatry at the University of Wisconsin, who has been aided by the Dalai Lama in his studies on the effects of meditation, reports that people can experience brain changes, including increases in gamma waves, in as little as two weeks of meditation practice.[40,41]

But you do need to make a commitment to meditate regularly. Research has shown that the more hours you spend meditating, the better you can sustain the kind of focused attention required for creative work. Davidson observes, "We've gotten this idea, in Western culture, that we can change our mental state by a once-a-week, forty-five minute intervention, which is complete cockamamy. Athletes and musicians train many hours every day. As a neuroscientist, I have to believe that engaging in compassion meditation every day for an hour each day would change your brain in important ways."[42]

WRITER'S APPLICATION:
WHAT KIND AND HOW MUCH?

There are a variety of meditation methods you can explore: Zen, Transcendental Meditation, compassionate meditation, mindfulness meditation, yoga, tai chi, qi gong. Meditation can be as simple as observing your breath and consistently bringing your attention back to your breathing when your mind wanders. Some people prefer moving meditations; swimming can be a great way to meditate (there is a built-in reminder to focus on regular breathing, after all).

In the Entering the Flow class I teach at the Loft, my students and I use focused breathing and mindfulness meditation as routes into the writer's trance. One of my Self-care practices is to meditate a half hour a day, six days a week. When my mediation practice is solid, I'm more relaxed, more creative and better able to focus on my writing for longer periods, so I'm more productive. I recognize that meditating for an hour a day would give me more profound benefits, but I also know that the half-hour commitment to sitting in mindfulness meditation is one I can and do consistently honor. An hour feels so big, I might be tempted to skip it far too often.

If you haven't meditated before, or if it's been awhile since you meditated, start small. Five minutes can be an amazingly long time to try to meditate when you first start. You might want to explore sample meditations in *The Blooming of a Lotus* or other books by Thich Nhat Hanh. Jon Kabat-Zinn, author of *Full Catastrophe Living* and one of Richard Davidson's research collaborators, has a collection of guided meditations available on CD.

INSIDE THE WRITER'S BRAIN:
THE POWER OF THE QUIET

In one of Davidson's studies, employees at a biotechnology company were divided into a test group who attended weekly classes in mindfulness meditation and meditated an hour a day for six days a week and a control group who did not attend classes or practice daily mediation. At the end of eight weeks, the test group not only reported feeling calmer, more focused and more creative, their brain scans were significantly different from their "before" scans taken at the beginning of the study and significantly different from the brain scans of the control group. Most notably, the test group increased the activity in their left prefrontal cortex.[43,44]

Previous studies demonstrate that people who consistently have more activity in their left prefrontal cortex than in their right prefrontal cortex tend to be "alert, energized, enthusiastic, and joyous, enjoying life more and having a greater sense of well-being."[45] On the other hand, these studies indicate that people who have a more active right prefrontal cortex tend to be more worried, anxious, sad and discontented with life. Greater activity in the left prefrontal cortex has also been shown to inhibit the amygdala, so we can reasonably assume that meditation will reduce the frequency, duration and intensity of limbic system takeovers, thus reducing writing resistance and leaving your creative cortex in the driver's seat more often.

Other than this asymmetrical increase in activity in the "optimistic" left prefrontal cortex, meditation tends to even out activity in the right and left hemispheres. It also increases the overall size of the prefrontal cortex and right anterior insula (areas that are related to focused attention and processing sensory data). Meditation reduces the levels of cortisol, the stress neurotransmitter. Cortisol is a leading cause of the negative effects of excessive stress, which include significantly reducing fluid intelligence (a.k. a. creative thinking) and impairing nearly every other cognitive function: mood, memory, learning, planning, self-control and motivation.[46]

If that's not enough to convince you to take up meditation, consider that stress also hampers the immune system, accelerates the aging process and interferes with your metabolism so that you're more likely to gain weight. Not only did meditation improve the immune systems of the meditators in Davidson's study, the degree of improvement could be predicted by the degree of increase of activity in the left prefrontal cortex.[47] Not surprisingly, study after study shows that the more hours you spend meditating, the more benefits you receive.

PLAY

Success Story: The Play's the Thing

The old saw about everything being grist for the mill when you're a writer is true. Your hobbies, passions and idiosyncrasies will inform your writing. For example, my novella features Nikki Wade, a ninety-two-year-old who realizes she isn't just losing her memories—they're being stolen and sold on the black market. This story draws on my memories of snorkeling in Hawaii, taking a zip-line tour of the jungle canopy in Costa Rica, visiting my grandmother when she lived in an assisted-living facility, playing countless games of cards with friends, working as an administrative assistant in the psychology department at the University of Minnesota, and a comment I made twenty years ago about traveling vicariously while looking at someone's vacation photos and thinking "Vicarious Vacations" would be a neat title for a science fiction story.

The fiction I'm working on now comes from the synchronistic combination of hearing a physicist explain his secret interest in time travel (not the topic a serious scientist trying to earn tenure advertises) and having recently taken up geocaching. I wondered what a GPS would be like if we could enter coordinates not just for latitude, longitude and altitude, but for the fourth dimension of time as well, and what a younger Nikki Wade would do if she could travel to parallel universes.

You never can tell when a piece of your life is going to spark a story element or poetic image. Who would have guessed that the field trip my class took to a brewery in Milwaukee when I was in grade school would be key research for a character in my novel who runs a distillery?

It's not surprising that I write about dogs in both my fiction and nonfiction since I'm as passionate (some say crazy) about dogs as I am about the brain. What's surprising is that the impetus to sign a contract for this book with Tarcher came at a dog agility trial. I was talking with a fellow competitor who mentioned she'd just returned home from a conference. We rarely talk about our occupations at trials—we're all dog geeks after all—but when I asked about the conference and discovered that this woman worked for Penguin Books, I mentioned that I was on the supply side of the business. And that was, as Bogie says in *Casablanca*, the beginning of a beautiful friendship.

Every experience you have has the potential to end up in your writing in some way. Everything you do is research. Your entire life is one gigantic field trip. However, don't expect the IRS to agree—I wouldn't even try to write off my trip to Hawaii as a business expense, although I will check with my tax advisor about deducting the entry fees for that dog trial. And don't try to get out of your share of household chores or social obligations either by telling your partner that staring at the ceiling or playing a game is work. Those household chores and social obligations also feed your creative work.

Play Is Serious Business

Despite what our Puritan forerunners asserted, play is not sinful. It is not a waste of time that could be better spent doing something "productive." It is not just a reward for hard work or an amusing diversion we squeeze into a busy schedule when we can.

Play is typically defined as a seemingly purposeless activity a person or other animal voluntarily engages in because the activity is inherently attractive. In other words, play is fun for fun's sake. The other elements that define play include the absence of time restrictions and expectations about outcomes, lack of concern about how others perceive us, and a willingness to improvise and entertain new possibilities.[48]

Some experts fear that we are losing creativity, cooperation and compassion because children and adults in industrialized countries don't engage in enough free play. Free play is defined as "imaginative and rambunctious fooling around that involves moving—jumping, running, wrestling—and aimless and creative actions."[49]

Play helps us figure out how to navigate our bodies through the physical world and how to navigate our psyches through the emotional and social world. We learn all kinds of important social skills in play: how to negotiate, argue constructively, act collaboratively, challenge ourselves to excel without trampling others, and how to lose gracefully and persevere.

Play is the natural way to learn, to practice, to rehearse without penalties. Play expands the imagination. Play is essential for creativity.

INSIDE THE WRITER'S BRAIN: THRIVING ON PLAY

According to Dr. Norman Doidge, author of *The Brain that Changes Itself*, "monotony undermines our dopamine and attentional systems crucial to maintaining brain plasticity."[50] Or in layperson's terms, "All work and no play makes Jack a dull boy."

Play gives us something to do with our big human brains. In fact, play has played a big part in the evolution of our big brains. Animals with comparatively larger brains for their body mass play more than animals with comparatively smaller brains. And the more playful behaviors a species typically engages in, the larger and more developed its frontal cortex and cerebellum are.[51]

Play is essential for brain development and helps the brain organize itself.[52] Play, especially active play, stimulates BDNF (a.k.a. Miracle-Gro for the brain) in the areas of the prefrontal cortex that make executive decisions.[53] As we have seen before, BDNF supports the growth of new neurons, encourages existing neurons to make new connections, and fights the effects of stress.

While some forms of play are solitary, play often gives us play-mates. This social interaction, which has been shown to be vital for brain development and well-being, may be part of why play improves mood. Research indicates that if we don't get enough play, we accumulate a play deficit, just as we accumulate a sleep deficit if we don't get enough sleep. While we don't know yet how harmful a play deficit is, we do know it makes us more pessimistic and unable to enjoy life.[54]

Because play promotes neurogenesis (growth of new neurons) throughout our lives, it keeps us young. People who play reduce their chances of getting Alzheimer's (by up to 63 percent in one study). Play postpones the onset of and mitigates the seriousness of age-related cognitive losses.[55] A variety of different forms of both physical and mental play keep the brain and the rest of the body flexible and strong. People who play are not only less likely to develop dementia, they're less likely to have heart disease.

Play keeps entropy at bay. As long as we play, we receive all the benefits of play. But if we stop playing, we stop developing, stop healing and re-creating our bodies and brains, stop engaging with others, stop truly enjoying life.

Play Is Creative

In addition to these direct brain benefits, play promotes creativity for a variety of other reasons. When we play, we make new associations and connections, imagine alternatives, play with novelty, and see metaphors and solutions.

We experiment without expectations, and those freewheeling experiments often lead to unexpected discoveries. As Dr. Stuart Brown points out in *Play*, "The first steam engine was a toy. So were the first airplanes. . . . When we are not up against life or death, trial and error brings out new stuff. We want to do this stuff not because we think that paper airplanes will lead to 747s. We do it because it's fun. And many years later, the 747 is born."[56]

Brown sees the creative impulse arising from the play impulse. "If we look at a life over time, and observe the origins of many artistic expressions, they are rooted in early play behavior that gets encouraged by natural talent and richness of opportunity in the environment. Watch a two-year-old who is drawn to music spontaneously dance to the beat of a summer band concert in the park. Fifteen years later, that kid may be a consummate pianist or just spend hours humming and strumming a guitar."[57]

And finally, because play is fun, it reduces stress and the limbic system takeovers triggered by stress. Anything that reduces stress has the net effect of improving our creativity.

WRITER'S APPLICATION: WHEN IS PLAY SELF-CARE AND WHEN IS PLAY PROCESS?

Experts group play into three categories: body play (active movement without time pressures or expectations), social play (interacting with others just for the fun of it) and object play (creating something with your hands with or without an anticipated end result, although if the goal is entirely economic, it's likely the activity is work rather than play).[58] Process is mostly likely to be object play or sometimes body play, although something like improvisational music or comedy that engages others could also be considered Process.

Ultimately, whether you call your play Self-care or Process is your call. Imposing rigid distinctions would only take the fun out of it.

As writers we need variety in our play: sometimes playing alone, sometimes with others, sometimes engaging in play with defined rules, sometimes engaging in play that is imaginatively free-form, sometimes moving our bodies, sometimes challenging our minds.

Instead of asking, "How much play is enough?" ask yourself, "How much play can I get away with?" Stay open to opportunities to turn any activity into play—you'll learn better, increase the health of your brain and the rest of your body and enjoy life more. Of course, some challenges must be endured for the sake of a desired outcome no matter how difficult or painful they are, but even these are easier when you maintain a playful attitude.

CHALLENGE: START YOUR SELF-CARE HABIT

You need to find a balance of activities and practices that keep you healthy and happy. Start with one of the five forms of Self-care that you're most interested in giving yourself. When you're consistently honoring your commitments to that form of Self-care, add another.

I suggest you copy and complete the Self-care Commitment Form below for each of the five forms of Self-care you're ready to commit to. (You can copy the PDF of this Self-care Commitment Form at http://BaneOfYourResistance.com/around-the-writers -block-forms/. Change the wording if necessary to make the form fit your commitments.) Just like you did for Process and Product Time, sign and date the form and ask a friend to sign and date it as your witness. Post the completed, signed and dated form in your calendar (or where you'll see it when making other appointments) to remind you that you have standing appointments with yourself.

My Self-care commitment to sleep is (number of) _____ hours a day, (number of) _____ days a week on (list the days) _____.

My Self-care commitment to exercise is to (indicate form of exercise) _____ (number of) _____ minutes a day, (number of) _____ days a week on (list the days) _____ _____ in the (indicate morning, afternoon or evening) _____ _____.

My Self-care commitment to focus is to (indicate how you will focus or what you will focus on) _____ _____ (number of) _____ minutes a day, (number of) _____ days a week on (list the days) _____ _____ in the (indicate morning, afternoon or evening) _____.

My Self-care commitment to meditation is (number of) _____ minutes a day, (number of) _____ days a week on (list the days) _____ in the (indicate morning, afternoon or evening) _____.

My Self-care commitment to play is to (indicate form of play) _____ (number of) _____ minutes a day, (number of) _____ days a week on (list the days) _____ _____ in the (indicate morning, afternoon or evening)_____.

Signed: _____ Date: _____
Witnessed by: _____ Date: _____

INQUIRY

"What am I doing to care for myself now? Do I treat myself as well as I treat others? If I had an extra hour a day, what could I do to become healthier, happier and more satisfied? Who else would benefit if I did that?"

Putting the Habits into Practice

6

RITUALS AND ROUTINES

Success Stories

Honoré de Balzac always put on a dressing gown that looked like a monk's robe before he wrote. Alexandre Dumas used different colors of paper and different pens for different kinds of writing; Saul Bellow had two typewriters—one for fiction, one for essays and criticism—that could never be interchanged. Charles Dickens moved the ornaments on his desk into a specific order before starting to write. Isabel Allende lights "candles for the spirits and the muses," surrounds herself with fresh flowers and incense, and meditates to open herself to her writing. Steven Pressfield wears his lucky work boots, drapes his lucky sweatshirt nearby, and positions his lucky cannon on a thesaurus pointed at his chair so "it can fire inspiration into me."

Few writing rituals make sense to anyone but the writer who

employs them. Some are even contradictory: Stephen King writes to loud rock and roll; May Sarton preferred eighteenth-century music only. Ernest Hemingway, Virginia Woolf, Lewis Carroll and Günter Grass all wrote standing up; Mark Twain, Truman Capote, Eudora Welty, Edith Wharton and William Styron all wrote lying down. John Cheever, Victor Hugo, John McPhee and Hope Dahle Jordan belong to what Ralph Keyes calls in *The Courage to Write* "the Bathrobe School"[1]; that is, they refrain from getting dressed until after they've finished the day's writing, so it's harder to leave the house to follow a distraction. Benjamin Disraeli, Anne Bernays and John Keats were all firm believers in the necessity of dressing professionally to write.

Despite a prevailing cultural bias against rituals as mere superstitions, writers have long known the power of ritual to reduce anxiety, increase confidence, and initiate and sustain their writing. As novelist John Edgar Wideman observed, "The variations are infinite, but each writer knows his or her version of the preparatory ritual must be exactly duplicated if writing is to begin, prosper."[2]

Why Are Writers So Superstitious?

In *The Courage to Write*, Ralph Keyes claims that writers use rituals to ease anxiety, pointing out that "ritualized behavior is common among those who do dangerous work."[3]

Twyla Tharp highlights the need for rituals when we are vulnerable. In *The Creative Habit*, she writes, "It's vital to establish some rituals—automatic but decisive patterns of behavior—at the beginning of the creative process, when you are most at peril of turning back, chickening out, giving up, or going the wrong way."[4] According to Tharp, ritual eliminates doubt, reassures us, puts us in motion, and gives us confidence to proceed.

Robert Olen Butler claims writers need rituals the way athletes do, to distract us from thinking too much about technique and how we do what we're doing. In *From Where You Dream*, Butler observes, "If the athlete begins to send the process into his head, he goes into a slump. He misses the basket, he misses that turn. Lights out. He drops the ball. I think, by the way, that's why athletes are so superstitious. Because if you believe that your current batting streak depends on wearing a pair of dirty socks, you're less likely to think it has to do with your technique. If it's technique, you think about it. If it's your socks, it's not rational. What superstitions do for the athlete is to irrationalize. And that's what you have to do as a writer; you have to irrationalize yourself somehow."[5]

Positioning a model cannon so it can fire inspiration into you, needing to wear your bathrobe or your lucky writer's hat, or using different-colored paper and pens for different kinds of writing are all pretty irrational. And at the same time, these rituals make perfect neurological sense.

INSIDE THE WRITER'S BRAIN:
NEURONS THAT FIRE TOGETHER,
WIRE TOGETHER

You may remember from chapter four that Hebb's Law states, "Neurons that fire together, wire together." In other words, when a group of neurons that process one movement, sensation or behavior are frequently activated at the same time that another group of neurons responsible for another movement, sensation or behavior are activated, those two groups of neurons will begin to make connections and fire simultaneously.

So if the neurons for smelling lemons are activated at the same time that the neurons you use when you're writing are activated, those two groups of neurons start to form a connection; they "wire together." Repetition reinforces this connection, so that eventually firing one set of neurons causes the other set to fire as well. The more you repeat the behaviors together and the more exclusive the behaviors are—you smell lemons only when writing—the more powerful the neural connection becomes. Eventually just smelling lemons will trigger the neurons used for writing and you'll "feel" like writing.

German playwright Friedrich Schiller applied this principle long before Hebb proposed his neuroplasticity concept. Schiller kept rotten apples in a drawer to keep his imagination alert. He used the association so much, he claimed he couldn't write without the odor. It may have had a secondary benefit of holding at bay anyone who would otherwise interrupt Herr Schiller's genius.

WRITER'S APPLICATION:
THAT REMINDS ME

Try this brain experiment—don't worry, you don't need a scalpel and a mirror, just a pen and a piece of paper.

Select an evocative scent, like the smell of fresh-baked bread. Remember the smell as vividly as you can. If it's a smell you can easily access, like vanilla or cinnamon, open a bottle of the real stuff and inhale. If you can't easily create the smell, don't worry, your memory will be enough. For a few moments close your eyes and focus on the smell or the memory of the smell.

Then list all the words that come to mind. You're going for quantity of words and ideas, not quality of sentences. If the smell of fresh-baked bread brings to mind all those Saturdays you spend with Aunt Martha kneading dough and baking bread, write:

Aunt Martha
Saturday mornings
Kneading
Sore shoulders
Damp towels
Flour on my hands
Butcher-block cutting board

Don't try to write sentences and paragraphs. Keep your mind free to float to other memories the smell of fresh-baked bread might evoke.

So go ahead and get a pen and paper, then select a scent. Here's a list of suggestions:

Vanilla
Bacon
Fire or smoke
Cinnamon
Fresh-cut grass
Wet wool sweater
Pumpkin pie
Coffee
Popcorn burned in the microwave
Mosquito repellent

Spend five or ten minutes creating your list of associations and memories.

So where did all these words, images and ideas come from? How does your brain do that? How can one smell evoke so many memories?

Experience Creates Connections

Smell is so provocative because the neurons for smell (and taste) run directly into the hippocampus, which is the center of long-term memory. Other senses are first intercepted and interpreted by the thalamus before being relayed to the hippocampus, which is why they are less powerful in evoking old memories.[6]

But any of the senses or a random thought can invoke memories because all the neurons in your brain are connected. Some connections are close and nearly instantaneous, like neural superhighways; others follow a more convoluted neural pathway and take longer to complete. And some connections are yet to be formed.

Experience changes the neural connections in your brain. These changes are not just limited to creating and storing new memories. In response to your life experiences, your brain has created and re-created, wired and rewired connections and neural pathways. So even though your brain is basically the same structure as other human brains, it is as individual as your fingerprints.

Your brain isn't a passive receptacle; it's not a soft-tissue equivalent of a bunch of filing cabinets that you just dump new information into when you experience or learn something new. Your brain rewires itself every time you experience something new. To be equivalent, a filing cabinet would have to spontaneously grow new drawers and reorganize the papers inside those drawers every time you added a file.

Right now, you may not have a writing ritual to comfort you, boost your confidence and keep you in motion. But you can change that. With several weeks of repetition, you can create a writing ritual out of just about any smell, taste, sound, sight, texture, movement or behavior by creating new neural connections. In other words, you can change your brain to make it more "writing friendly."

You could create a neural connection between wearing a lucky writer's cap and writing, the taste of lemon drops and writing, the smell of stinky socks and writing, or, if you're Friedrich Schiller, the smell of rotten apples and writing.

Let's assume you prefer lemon drops to getting hat hair or the smell of stinky socks and rotten apples. If you were to eat a lemon drop every time you wrote for several weeks, your brain would create new connections between those two groups of neurons. According to Hebb's Law, the neurons for eating lemon drops would wire up with the neurons for writing. The smell or taste of lemon would not only trigger your "lemon drop neurons" to fire, it would also trigger your "writing neurons" to fire.

The more often we associate a ritual with writing, and the more exclusively we associate the ritual only with writing, the more effectively the presence of the ritual triggers the "writing neurons" to fire.

INSIDE THE WRITER'S BRAIN: RITUALS BY ANY OTHER NAME

It's certainly true that ritualized routines comfort us. The familiar is soothing. No one has done research on this specifically, but I strongly suspect that the familiarity of a writing ritual relaxes us enough to keep the cortex in control or to cause the RAS to flip control from the limbic system to the cortex.

Even if the ritual isn't enough to keep the amygdala and the rest of the limbic system from acting up when you start writing, you can still follow the ritual into your writing. Remember, when the limbic system is in control, your actions follow the instinctual fight-or-flight response and what you've learned in repeated training. As you repeat a ritual, you're training yourself to take that action automatically. Repeated neural patterns become easier to trigger without conscious thought—remember Pavlov's dogs.

Like a pilot trained to respond to emergencies, we can train ourselves to keep writing. Behaviors that are this ingrained are considered automatic processes, which can be used by both the cortex and the limbic system.

CHALLENGE: PICK A RITUAL, ANY RITUAL AT ALL

Identify the rituals and routines in your life. For example, do you brush your teeth every morning? I put my glasses on only after I've taken my morning vitamins and allergy pill, so I know that if I have my glasses on, I've taken my pills that day. And while writing this book, I always started my writing with a whiff of vanilla extract.

Identify any rituals, routines or almost-routines you have in your writing life. Do you always check your email before you write? (This may not be the best routine, and you might want to transfer the association to start writing with another activity that won't distract you as much or as long.) Do you often have a cup of latte or tea when you write? What behaviors have you learned to associate with writing? If you don't have a writing ritual or routine, develop one. If you do, consider how you could tweak those routines to make it easier to start writing.

Recall that smell signals, unlike other sensory experiences, do not have to pass through the thalamus before going directly to the hippocampus or other higher areas of the brain. Because smell has direct access to the amygdala, it is a powerful trigger for emotions, which in turn affect motivation.[7] Adding a scent component to your writing ritual makes brain sense.

Stop in the Middle Of

Supposedly, Hemingway stopped his daily writing in the middle of a sentence so he'd know where to start the next day. Hemingway's ritual of stopping in the middle was an ending ritual that led him straight into the next day's opening ritual. He advised, "The best way is always to stop when you are going good and when you know what will happen next. If you do that every day . . . you will never be stuck. Always stop while you are going good and don't think about it or worry about it until you start to write the next day. That way your subconscious will work on it all the time."

James Thurber attests to the observation that writers are working even when it looks like we aren't. "I never quite know when I'm not writing. Sometimes my wife comes up to me at a party and says, 'Dammit, Thurber, stop writing.' She usually catches me in the middle of a paragraph."

Never-ending writing may sound ideal; your unconscious keeps turning the pieces of the puzzle over and over until something clicks into place and voilà, you have another of those exciting and satisfying "aha" moments. But there are times when we need help to stop writing.

Despite having solid writing habits that had sustained her for years, Jackie W. struggled to keep working when she started to write about her infant son's death in her book about complicated grief. "It's hard to write about what happened," she told me in a coaching session, "but I knew it would be and I know it'll be worth it. The problem is that I can't stop thinking about those awful memories. I feel drained and emotionally hungover. It's like the past is leaking out and staining the rest of my life."

Jackie already had a writing ritual: she lit a candle and asked for spiritual guidance and protection in her writing. I suggested she modify the ritual slightly to include declaring—out loud or in writing—that she was willing to explore those memories during her writing session and only during her writing session. I also suggested she add a closing ritual to declare that she was no longer willing to entertain those memories, ask for protection for the rest of the day, and then blow out the candle. Adding the closing ritual didn't make the memories less painful, but it did allow Jackie to restrict the memories to when she was willing to work with them. It freed her from dragging the emotional baggage around for the rest of the day.

A closing ritual creates a container for painful memories and material. It also creates a neural pattern to shift your thinking and behavior. A closing ritual complements and completes the opening ritual. Together, an opening and closing ritual bookend the writing session and help us compartmentalize our work. When memoirists are working with painful memories, when fiction writers are writing the dark moments or following the alarming twists of the antagonist's mind, when any writer is working with challenging, painful material, that compartmentalization is what allows us to do the work at all.

It's been said that the purpose of art is to comfort the disturbed and disturb the comfortable. As artists, we have to be willing to go deep, to explore the underside of our society and our own psyches. As human beings, we need to know we don't have to dwell in that darkness 24/7. We need to know we can stop. We need a ritual to signal, especially to our image-focused right hemisphere, that we are stopping.

CHALLENGE: RITUAL REVERSE

If you use a ritual or routine to get your writing started, think about a way to reverse it to create a logical ending ritual. If you don't have a ritual, consider what patterns you would like to use as an opening and closing routine. Even when the writing you're doing isn't challenging, it's useful to know when to stop writing and rejoin the world. That way, your partner won't have to nudge you in the ribs the way Mrs. Thurber did.

INSIDE THE WRITER'S BRAIN: USE IT OR LOSE IT

The human brain is plastic, not fluid; it is capable of profound change, but it is also remarkably consistent.

Myelin is the source of the brain's consistency. In a healthy brain, myelin never disappears. Once a neural pathway is insulated, it stays insulated, which is why the habits we wish we never formed are so frustratingly persistent.[8] After all, myelin is fatty tissue, and we all know how difficult it is to get rid of fat. (I suppose this means it would be accurate to say that the term "fathead" applies to anyone who is entrenched in old patterns of thought and behavior.)

On the other hand, with focused repetition, the brain can create new neural pathways and connections. Because they don't lose myelin, the old pathways are still there, but they can be superseded by new patterns. Neuroplasticity is a double-edged sword. Because your brain is flexible enough to create new neural pathways for habits and routines you want to cultivate, it's also flexible enough to replace pathways you stop using. "Use it or lose it" is the corollary to Hebb's Law.

Routines you practice will remain; routines you ignore will fade, especially if they are relatively new routines (with less myelination). You can't leave your writing for prolonged periods without feeling that you're starting over almost from scratch. If you don't keep employing the neurons you've enlisted as your writing neurons, they'll go work for someone else, performing a different routine.

INQUIRY

"How can I design and practice rituals to support myself as a writer, an artist and a human being?"

RECORD AND REWARD

Success Story

Even though she'd published one book, writer and playwright Annette D. wanted to improve her writing habits. She knew she needed structure and frequently felt overwhelmed by the choice of several projects to focus on. She realized that shifting between projects was often a way to avoid making a commitment to any one of them. "Time seemed to slip away with nothing to show for it but good intentions to do better tomorrow."

When Annette decided to practice Process, Self-care and Product Time, she discovered that checking in each week with other writers about what she intended to do and what she actually did made the commitment real. Recording her progress in a log and rewarding herself when she honored her promises helped even more. And sticking to her commitments to Process, Self-care and

Product Time allowed Annette to create structure out of what felt like a vast and swirling ocean of ideas and projects.

"Like any new habit, it was difficult at first. I had an especially hard time making room to pursue some sort of artistic process practice. I tried lots of things—listening intently to music I wanted to explore, drawing tropical fish, journal pages, dance practice—mixing it up to make Process a form of creative cross-training. I still find that Process is the hardest of the three practices to pull off each week, but I do it because I made the commitment and because, like Pavlov's dog, I look forward to my reward."

Adopting the idea of rewarding herself was also difficult. Annette couldn't think of anything that motivated her or felt like a worthy reward. When she admitted to herself that she was motivated by money, Annette started paying herself a dollar every time she honored one of her commitments, setting the money aside in an old check box.

"I had to literally pay myself with dollar bills; otherwise the reward was too abstract, like the money wasn't really there, or I should donate it or save it for something 'more important.' Now my challenge is to spend it on myself so it really is a reward."

One of Annette's favorite rewards was spending the money she earned doing her daily practices on a kayaking adventure trip. She also used it to buy special earrings that were more expensive than what she would usually buy for herself. "That's been surprisingly reinforcing. I wear them almost every day, and I see them, I like them and I'm proud that I earned them. They remind me that I am a writer.

"It's been well over a year that I've been this disciplined and structured about my creative life, and I have a new full-length play as the result. I don't think I would have gotten this far if I hadn't used this system of tracking and rewards."

Writer's Log: Stardate 2012

Keeping a writer's journal means different things to different writers: a way to practice the craft of writing, a repository of great ideas, a log of what you've researched, a library of opening and closing lines and snatches of dialogue, a place to dredge up memories. Young writers keep journals in the hope that someday fans and English lit majors will want to know how they worked; elder writers keep journals in the certainty that memory is fleeting and fickle.

No doubt you'll find benefits in any kind of writer's journal you keep. I've observed that the clients and students who keep daily entries about what they do for each of the three practices of Process, Self-care and Product Time are more consistent in honoring their commitments, build sustainable habits faster, and are more satisfied with their performance and experience than those who don't keep track. The log can be as simple as a table where you record your commitments for each of the three practices and make daily entries about what you actually do for each. (You can find a PDF of a Three Habits Tracking Table at http://BaneOfYourResistance.com/around-the-writers-block-forms/.)

Emerging novelist and memoirist L. Nygaard credits tracking

the three practices with developing her regular writing routine. She observed, "I found that tracking what I did for the practices was almost as important as doing the practices themselves." As they became integral to her writing life and Process, Self-care and Product Time were as routine as brushing her teeth in the morning, recording her daily progress became less necessary. "But when my routine changes or my practices waffle, I return to a weekly tracking form to record each day's commitments, targets, and accomplishments."

Like L. Nygaard, I have enough history with my habits that I no longer need to record what I do for Process and Self-care. But I

	Monday 4/23/12	Tuesday 4/24/12	Wednesday 4/25/12	Thursday 4/26/12	Friday 4/27/12	Saturday 4/28/12	Sunday 4/29/12
Process (Commitment: 15 minutes a day, 5 days a week)	Morning pages 20 min.	Morning pages 15 min.	Colored 17 min.	Played harmonica 15 min.	Morning pages 20 min.	n/a (no commitment today)	Collage 25 min.
Self-care (Commitment: 30 minutes a day, 6 days a week)	Yoga 30 min.	Workout 45 min.	Yoga 30 min.	Workout 40 min.	Meditate 20 min.	Walk 60 min.	n/a
Product Time (Commitment: 15 minutes a day, 5 days a week)	Research for novel 15 min.	Query letter 18 min.	Drafting 1 hour	Drafting 15 min.	Research 20 min.	n/a	n/a

do keep detailed records for my Product Time. The table I use includes columns for:

- Date
- Intended target time (when I intend to start and how long I intend to work)
- Intended target task (what I intend to work on)
- Actual time (when I actually started and how long I actually worked)
- What I actually worked on
- Reward
- How I feel about the day's effort
- What I want to focus on next time

(You can find a PDF of a Product Time Tracking Table at http://BaneOfYourResistance.com/around-the-writers-block -forms/.)

You might notice that I don't log my commitment to Product Time; this is because it is an unwavering fifteen minutes a day, five days a week, Monday through Friday.

I tally weekly totals for intended target time and actual time and calculate the percentage of the target I actually worked. Day to day, I don't worry about target time compared to actual time, but I do pay attention to the weekly percentages.

INSIDE THE WRITER'S BRAIN:
"ATTENTION MUST BE PAID"

The brain changes in response to what we pay attention to. More important, the brain does not change if we're not paying attention. When monkeys are trained to detect subtle changes in the vibration frequencies of an object fluttering on one fingertip, the portion of their somatosensory cortex that corresponds to that finger increases significantly. This is classic neuroplasticity at work. However, when monkeys are exposed to the same object fluttering on a fingertip, but are distracted by sounds, their somatosensory cortex doesn't change.[1]

Dr. Jeffrey Schwartz observes in *The Mind & the Brain*, "When stimuli *identical* to those that induce plastic changes in an attending brain are instead delivered to a nonattending brain, there is no induction of cortical plasticity. Attention, in other words, must be paid."[2]

If you want to form a new habit, it's vital to focus your attention on the new behavior. The more you pay attention to the new writing habits you want to develop, the more plastic your brain can be in acquiring those new habits. Recording what you do for Process, Self-care and Product Time in a log is an excellent way to pay attention.

As the Egyptian pharaohs used to say, "So let it be written, so let it be done."

Benefits of Tracking

Recording also increases your awareness, motivation and the likelihood of repeating the desired behavior. For example, according to the *American Journal of Preventive Medicine*, dieters who consistently record what they eat lose up to twice as much weight as those who don't keep a food diary.[3]

Keeping a writer's log will help you maintain focus and give yourself full credit for what you do. Remember, the most effective way to evaluate Product Time is not by how many words you produce, but simply by whether or not you show up when you say you will. When you're struggling in Incubation or with a challenging rewrite, it can seem that you're not making progress. This is when your writer's log can reassure you that you are doing what you need to do. When you have several months of entries, you can look back on other times you struggled and see what helped you find a solution.

It's too easy to lose track of all the work you do on a writing project, especially since losing track of time is one of the hallmarks of the flow state we all want to achieve. Yet, in *Creativity*, Mihaly Csikszentmihalyi identifies immediate feedback as one of the nine components required for the flow state and observes that those who keep doing creative work are those who can give themselves feedback.[4] Tracking is one way to give yourself feedback and acknowledge your efforts.

It also allows you to compare what you intend to do with what you actually do and address any potential problems before they get too big. You may not have a precise match between your intention and your actual activity, and most of the time that's okay. If you have the freedom to change your schedule at the last minute or shift your focus to follow a new intriguing idea, why not enjoy it? But with that freedom comes the challenge of not only motivating yourself, but also holding yourself accountable.

To do that, you need precise information, not just a vague sense of, "I put in a lot of hours this week, I think. Except for Tuesday, or was it Wednesday, when I had to run errands?" Logging in your start and stop times will keep you honest. Comparing the total number of hours you targeted to the total number of hours you worked for the week lets you know whether you should adjust your efforts to meet your goals, modify your target estimates to fit reality, or give yourself a bonus reward in addition to daily rewards.

Including a column for Reward in your tracking log will remind you to give yourself the small, daily rewards that reinforce the routine tasks of showing up, opening the files and just getting started. Once you get into the writing, the challenge of solving the puzzle is its own reward, but the daily rewards support the mechanical steps that make it possible to get to the intrinsic rewards.

Tracking also focuses your attention on how you feel about your writing every day. As you'll see in the case of a British naval officer's brush with disaster, below, emotions are valuable information from the limbic system. When we notice how we feel, we can gain conscious awareness of what our limbic system already knows: that something significant is on the horizon.

INSIDE THE WRITER'S BRAIN:
WHEN THE LIMBIC SYSTEM
IS RIGHT ON TARGET

During Desert Storm, British naval officer Lieutenant Commander Michael Riley of the HMS *Gloucester* was responsible for monitoring the radar reports of the airspace surrounding the Allied fleet. Early one morning, Riley noticed a blip headed toward the fleet from the Kuwaiti coast that he just didn't like. If the blip was an Iraqi missile, it was on course to destroy the USS *Missouri*, an American battleship with hundreds of sailors aboard. But the blip looked just like an American fighter jet, and the American pilots routinely turned off their electronic identification system so they couldn't be tracked by Iraqi antiaircraft missiles. The only piece of equipment that could give Riley the information he needed, the blip's altitude, was temporarily offline. Riley simply could not know for sure what this blip was. But he had to make a decision, and fast.[5]

What was going on in Riley's mind was probably something along the lines of, "Is it one of ours? If it is, and I give the order to shoot it down, I'll kill two American pilots. But if it's not, hundreds aboard the *Missouri* will die. I have a really bad feeling about this."

What was going on in Riley's brain was that his limbic system had detected a deviation in a pattern that his cortex couldn't detect. It would be months later before a psychologist studying battlefield decision making would notice that the blip that worried Riley appeared on his radar screen a mere eight seconds later than an American fighter jet would have appeared. When his limbic system detected this eight-second deviation, Riley's dopamine-releasing neurons stopped firing. It was the decrease in dopamine that gave Riley the bad feeling and that pinged his intuition enough for him to give the order to fire.

The limbic system is not only "to blame" for limbic system takeovers, it is also the source of valuable information the cortex can't perceive. The limbic system does not include the language centers, so we don't have words when the limbic system detects something significant. Emotions are the limbic system's only language. And since the limbic system knows things the cortex doesn't, paying attention to how we feel about our writing (or blips on the radar screen or anything else) is our smartest move. Of course, you need your cortex to interpret emotions and plan a course of action, but you can trust that your emotions are there for a reason.

WRITER'S APPLICATION: TRACK IT

I recommend you track Process, Self-care and Product Time for at least six months while you're developing these habits. You can copy the sample table for tracking the three habits shown on page 151 or incorporate your own tracking system into whatever date-book or calendar app you use. You can even post a chart on your office wall and give yourself gold stars or other stickers every time you honor a commitment. Many students admit with a mix of embarrassment and defiance that the gold stars that motivated them in grade school still have the power to engage them as adults. The key, as you'll see below, is that they are the ones giving themselves the gold stars, not some external authority figure.

Plan on keeping a detailed Product Time log for the rest of your writing career. Refer to the categories listed on page 152 to design your own table, and modify them to fit your needs. (You can copy the PDF of the table I use for Product Time tracking at http://BaneOfYourResistance.com/around-the-writers-block -forms/.)

It Pays to Pay Yourself

Children's writer Peter Pearson once described himself as a "'fraidy-cat writer who learned to knuckle down and face the blank page" by consistently paying himself for his writing success. Peter puts a gold dollar coin in small wooden chest every day after the day's writing is done.

"My great-great-grandfather made this sewing box, but I use it as my writing treasure chest. When I look inside, I see everything I've ever done and it gives me hope. When things seem impossible, I just crack the lid open, peer in, and think, 'I've done this before. I can do it again.' There's nothing like a chest full of gold coins to get the blood going."

Peter is about to earn his MFA, has completed a novel draft, and is working on picture books. He credits a large part of his success to the three habits and to consistently rewarding himself for showing up.

If you want to write more often and more effectively, putting yourself on the payroll, like Annette D., Peter Pearson and a lot of other writers, is a good first step.

INSIDE THE WRITER'S BRAIN: WHY REWARDS WORK

When a person gets what she/he sees as a reward, the brain secretes two neurotransmitters: dopamine and acetylcholine. Dopamine is the feel-good neurotransmitter that brings pleasure, energy and confidence. Acetylcholine helps the brain pay attention to what has just happened and form a memory of the experience. Dopamine also reinforces memory by strengthening the connections between the neurons that were active when the reward was received. Together dopamine and acetylcholine essentially say, "Pay attention to this; this is an experience worth remembering and repeating." Because they activate the limbic dopamine system, rewards make learning easier.[6]

Interestingly, the anterior cingulate, an area of the brain that is key to self-motivation and to modifying behavior to correct errors (which is why some neuroscientists call this the "oh, shit" circuit), lights up like a Christmas tree when a reward is anticipated as well as when it's received.[7]

However, in *Drive: The Surprising Truth About What Motivates Us*, Daniel Pink demonstrates how the commonsense principle that rewards improve performance applies only for routine, step-by-step tasks (algorithmic tasks). Study after study has shown that for tasks that require creative thinking to find a novel solution (heuristic tasks), rewards actually impair performance. And the bigger the reward, the bigger the impairment.[8]

Since writing is primarily heuristic, it might seem that we simply should avoid rewards. Indeed a lot of my students and clients have an intuitive understanding about this when they insist, "Writing should be its own reward." The trouble is that these are the same writers who are struggling with the frustration and confusion of not understanding why they aren't doing the writing they want and love to do. They have the intrinsic motivation to write, but are blocked by resistance. In these cases, I've found that rewards can be thoughtfully employed to reduce resistance, particularly when the focus is on, and the reward is given for, effort rather than outcomes.

So before we leap from the unthinking commonsense assumption that rewards are always good to the misguided conclusion that rewards are always bad, let's look more closely at when and why rewards have a negative impact on heuristic tasks, and when and why they might have a positive effect on some aspects of our writing.

What Rewards Do to Creativity

Rewards narrow both the depth and breadth of our thinking to, "What do I have to do to get the reward?" which precludes the kind of creative thinking that comes from open-ended questions like, "How about . . ." "Why not . . ." and "What else . . ."

Rewards also reduce or destroy intrinsic motivation, which is essential for creativity. After reviewing three decades of research studies, Edward Deci concluded, "Careful consideration of reward effects reported in 128 experiments lead to the conclusion that tangible rewards tend to have a substantially negative effect on intrinsic motivation."[9]

Or as Mark Twain put it, "Work consists of whatever a body is *obliged* to do, and . . . Play consists of whatever a body is not obliged to do."

Rewards send the message, "I know this isn't something you're going to like to do, so I promise to give you something you will like if you do this task." You might think that when we're promised a reward for something we want to do anyway, we'd be smart enough to just take the reward and think, "Ha, got you fooled. I enjoyed the task and got the reward." And in some situations we can do that, but the presence of a reward frequently changes our perception of the task from play to work, just as Mr. Twain predicts.

But it's important to note that rewards have this negative effect on intrinsic motivation only when they are contingent, that is, when they are some form of, "If you do this, then you get that." Unexpected rewards that are a celebration after the fact, the "Now that you've made this effort, here's a reward" variety, actually boost future creativity.

Contingent, if-then rewards limit autonomy, one of the three key sources of intrinsic motivation. In one study, Teresa Amabile, one of the world's leading researchers on creativity, asked twenty-three professional artists to submit ten commissioned works and ten noncommissioned works, selected by the artists at random. Not surprisingly, the artists reported that they had felt more constrained when working on the commissioned pieces. Furthermore, a panel of artists and curators, who were unaware of the purposes of the study, consistently found the commissioned works less creative than the noncommissioned works.[10]

But Amabile's study also discovered that when artists saw the commission as enabling them to do something interesting and exciting, or when they thought the commission provided useful information or feedback, artists produced works that the panel of judges considered as creative as the noncommissioned work.

As long as creative people can keep their focus on the creative task instead of the reward, the reward doesn't have to impair their performance. In *The Owner's Manual for the Brain*, Dr. Pierce J. Howard observes, "The highest creativity occurs when we discover the need for a creative response ourselves and choose to contribute independent of any possible external constraints. When external constraints, such as deadlines, rewards or punishers, are imposed on a personally desirable task, creativity can still flourish if we are able to cognitively minimize the constraints. When we are unable to forget about them, creativity suffers."[11]

Paradoxically, artists who are least interested in extrinsic rewards and who pursue art for the challenge and joy of creating are more likely to get both the intrinsic satisfaction and the extrinsic rewards of success, recognition and money.[12]

What we don't know is what happens when rewards that are usually extrinsic (cash, bonuses, food treats, etc.) are provided to a writer by the writer herself. We can assume that giving yourself a reward wouldn't decrease your sense of autonomy, although it may limit the depth and breadth of your thinking. As far as I can tell from my investigations, no one has researched the question of whether self-rewards necessarily limit creativity. Until more research is available, I suggest you be wary of rewards offered by authority figures, focus on the intrinsic rewards of writing itself, and find ways to reward yourself for performing routine tasks.

What Rewards Do for Routine Tasks

Rewards do increase the speed and effectiveness of performance in routine tasks with clear solutions. And nothing can reduce intrinsic motivation in a task that doesn't have any intrinsic interest to begin with.[13]

No matter how much you love the challenge and thrill of discovery you get when you solve a writing puzzle, there will always be some routine tasks that simply have to be done. Writing an effective query letter, for example, is creatively challenging, but once you've written it, copying and pasting it into an email or shoving it in an envelope is routine. So are keeping track of what pieces you've submitted to which editors, updating research notes and financial records, filing, and the other administrivia needed to run an office. Finding ways to reward yourself for tackling these routine tasks will make those tasks, well, more rewarding.

And no matter how much we love writing as a whole, no matter how closely what we're working on reflects our passion and purpose, each of us prefers some stages of the creative process more than others. Don't bother looking for rewards for the tasks that are part of the stages that intrigue you and provide their own intrinsic satisfaction. The stages that don't rock your world are better candidates for rewards.

If you love a particular part of writing and you consistently show up to do that part, don't mess it up by imposing a reward system on it. But for the stages you struggle with and the parts of the process that make you crinkle your nose, rewards can get you going and keep you moving. If you're feeling resistant to a part of the writing you usually can't wait to get started on, explore options for rewarding yourself to break the inertia. If you have difficulty getting yourself to your writing space and getting started, give yourself a small reward just for showing up and another small reward for starting (by opening your notebook, computer file or research, for example).

CHALLENGE: ONE SIZE DOESN'T FIT ALL

Rewards are individual. My big reward might be a ho-hum reward or no reward at all for you. Giving a reward that isn't valued by the person receiving it is a waste of energy and can actually demotivate the receiver. You need to think about what is truly rewarding for you and what rewards you find mildly, moderately and strongly appealing.

Timing is also crucial. To maximize the brain benefit of a reward, it needs to be provided at the same time or immediately after the desired behavior. That way, the dopamine and acetylcholine are associated with the desired behavior. If you delay the reward to think about what to give yourself, you dissipate the effectiveness of the reward.

This is why you need a list of potential rewards in advance. Prepare a list of ten small rewards, ten medium rewards, and ten large rewards. For example, to me a small reward is fifty cents dropped into a metal box that sits on my desk; a medium reward is a single piece of high-quality chocolate; a large reward is jewelry or a nonessential piece of clothing (I gave myself a top-quality rain jacket to wear at agility trials when I completed chapter five) or guilt-free time off to take a trip.

INSIDE THE WRITER'S BRAIN: THE RIGHT KIND OF ATTENTION

Dr. Carol Dweck, psychologist at Stanford University, conducted a study with four hundred New York City fifth graders who were given puzzles and then were either praised for their intelligence by a researcher saying, "You must be smart at this [*sic*]," or praised for their effort by a researcher saying, "You must have worked really hard." The students were then given the option of working with easy puzzles, similar to the ones they'd just solved, or a more challenging set of puzzles that they could learn a lot from. Most of the students who were praised for their intelligence chose the easier set of puzzles, while 90 percent of the students praised for their effort chose the more challenging set.[14]

When Dweck gave these fifth-grade students a third test designed for eighth graders, the ones who were praised for their intelligence were easily discouraged and saw their mistakes as failures. Furthermore, when they took a fourth test at the same difficulty level as the first test, their performance decreased by 20 percent. Their experience of failure on the third test impaired their ability. On the other hand, students who were praised for their effort were engaged in and worked hard on the eighth-grade-level test and actually increased their performance on the final test by 30 percent.

Praising students for their intelligence rewards their performance and focuses their attention on the outcome; praising students for their effort rewards their willingness to try and focuses attention on the process. Students praised for effort have greater intrinsic motivation to challenge themselves to continue to learn and develop. They are better prepared to respond positively to situations where they don't have all the answers.

Recording what you do for Product Time, Self-care and Process is a way of focusing your attention on the effort you're making. It can be your way of telling yourself, "I'm really giving this a good effort," on a daily basis. In fact, saying that out loud is one way to reward yourself. Recording is also a handy antidote for our culture's focus on results only. So many writers are discouraged when friends and family invariably ask about outcomes: "Have you published anything?" "Did you get a contract yet?" or "Finished that novel yet?" Tracking gives you the information you need to say something like, "I'm doing great. I show up for my writing when I say I will and I'm meeting 75 percent of my Big Audacious Targets."

Your friends and family don't ask about outcomes to undermine you; they ask about outcomes because that's our cultural bias (despite how unhelpful Dweck and other researchers have shown this to be). Every time you respond by talking about your effort, you're training the people you care about to shift to a perspective that will better support your intrinsic motivation and theirs.

INSIDE THE WRITER'S BRAIN: STROKES, MONKEYS, AND OVEN MITTS

When a person has a stroke, some neurons in the affected area of the brain are killed outright, some are injured. Some of the injured neurons will heal and some of the killed neurons will be replaced. Stroke patients can recover some or nearly all of their former abilities; how much they recover depends on the severity of the stroke, the speed of medical intervention and other factors.

However, as mentioned in chapter two, if a stroke victim gives up trying to use whatever part of the body—hand, arm, leg, etc.— was incapacitated by the stroke, the healing neurons won't be challenged to do what they used to do. Because neurons are too precious to go unused, they'll be recruited to perform some other function. So a hand, for example, that was initially incapacitated by a stroke continues to be nonfunctioning, not because of the stroke damage, but because the person stopped using that hand. The muscles atrophy, but more important, the corresponding area of the brain atrophies. Dr. Edward Taub calls this "learned non-use," a phenomena he first noted in his research with monkeys.

Taub is perhaps best-known and most highly regarded for developing a profoundly improved treatment for stroke patients. At the Taub Therapy Clinic, patients wear oven mitts and slings to keep the hand or arm not affected by a stroke immobilized so they are forced to use the hand or arm that was affected by the stroke. Patients play games you'd normally see toddlers playing—pushing pegs into holes, picking up pennies or beans—to relearn how to use the affected limb. For hours of daily practice, patients are encouraged to focus on incremental improvements and congratulated for behaviors that approximate the desired end result, a technique behaviorists call "shaping."[15]

In previous research with monkeys that had had one arm partially paralyzed, Taub observed that classical conditioning of providing a reward if the monkey used the affected arm didn't work. Taub's monkeys made much better progress when he provided a reward "not only for successfully reaching for the food, but for making the first, most modest gesture toward it."[16] In other words, Taub's monkeys responded to the shaping technique.

WRITER'S APPLICATION: TAKE THE GLOVES OFF AND PUT THE MITTS ON

Deep-seated writing resistance may be a kind of learned non-use. Writing injuries, like sports injuries, are an unfortunate but frequent part of the game. From the time we entered grade school, we were publicly and privately corrected, rejected, criticized, embarrassed, unappreciated, censored and ignored. Fortunately, we were also praised, celebrated and held up for public approval, or we would have given up writing altogether. Some writers are more resilient than others, some writers are luckier than others, but we've all been injured in one way or another in the past.

Withdrawing is a natural response to physical or emotional pain, but a temporary withdrawal can become permanent if the writer doesn't have the opportunity, encouragement and grit to try again. Injured writers, like injured athletes, naturally and unconsciously compensate for the injury—we stop writing dialogue or avoid certain constructions or stop sharing writing with particular audiences. And just as with physical injuries, these compensating moves can interfere with full recovery.

If we are unwilling or unable to accept and celebrate imperfect performance while recovering, we may give up trying that skill or technique. When the neural pathway for a particular writing skill goes unused for too long, that is, when the neurons are not firing together, they no longer wire together. If we stop using a particular ability, we lose that ability.

Perhaps one of the reasons extrinsic rewards impair performance in creative tasks is because they're used in a classic conditioning approach, where the reward is given only when the behavior is exactly the desired end result. Heuristic tasks are typically more complicated than routine tasks, so it's not surprising that it takes more time and trials to achieve the desired end result. When we take the focus off the end result and apply a shaping technique, where we give rewards for approximate behavior, we may see that extrinsic rewards can be an effective part of motivating and improving performance in creative tasks.

So how do we put on the oven mitts as writers? How can we shape our behavior to recover atrophied writing skills and gain new ones? The first step is to assess the injury and identify which skills and potentials have atrophied over time. But if, like Aimee the French amnesiac, we're affected by slight injuries we don't recall, how do we challenge ourselves to reclaim and regain those skills? And how do we tell the difference between a skill, technique or genre we abandoned because of an injury and those we're simply not interested in?

To identify what we've abandoned and need to reclaim, we need to look to the wisdom of our emotions. Aimee knew something was wrong because she was afraid to shake her doctor's hand. She wasn't just uninterested in shaking hands—her mouth got dry, her palms sweated, and her stomach clenched. To take the first step of identifying and assessing the injury, we need to ask ourselves and seriously ponder questions like:

- What am I afraid to write?
- What do I believe I could never write? Have I ever tested that assumption?
- What do I most regret not writing? When I'm in my eighties, what will I have the most regret about not pursuing?
- What do I wish I could write? What would be so wonderful, so cool, so freaking good that I can't really believe I could write it?
- What writers do I admire, even idolize, and what do they have that I wish I had?
- When I fantasize, what awards do I imagine myself winning—a Pulitzer, a Newbury, a Hugo, a Pushcart or an O. Henry?

The second step (and the third step and the fourth step and so on) is to practice the skill we want to acquire and to reward ourselves for making, as Taub said, "the first, most modest gesture toward it." In other words, we shape our writing behavior. We put in the 10,000 hours of practice that Malcolm Gladwell says we need to acquire mastery. And we put in those 10,000 hours by showing up for fifteen minutes at a time and rewarding ourselves for every small step along the way.

Puppies and Teeter-totters: Shaping Behavior

Years ago, I used shaping and rewards to train my puppy Blue to navigate a teeter-totter and other obstacles found in the sport of dog agility. Most of what dogs do in agility training are natural behaviors—running, jumping, climbing—but the teeter-totter is not. The teeter is weighted so that one end stays on the ground. The dog has to run up the board, pause at just the right place where her weight causes the board to tip, and ride the board until the up end touches the ground.

If I had lured Blue into walking the teeter-totter by putting treats in front of her nose to direct her or putting treats on the teeter-totter—in other words, if I had used contingent, if-then rewards—Blue probably would have learned that even though the teeter was scary, it offered rewards. But she would not want to play with the teeter if there weren't any treats around. Instead, my trainer showed me how I could use rewards to help Blue learn that the teeter-totter was interesting, not scary, and that interacting with it was fun, not work. I praised Blue and gave her treats, but I never asked her to do anything. She initiated all her movements;

I just rewarded the ones that were close to a series of behaviors we were looking for (rewarding approximate behaviors).

At first, I clicked the clicker and gave Blue a small treat anytime she looked at the teeter-totter. This made the teeter interesting and a place where good things happened, so Blue started looking for it when we went to class. After several short training sessions, I upped the ante just a little. I continued to click and give Blue a reward anytime she approached the teeter-totter, but stopped giving so many rewards for just looking at the board. When Blue sniffed or touched the teeter, she got extra treats.

I continued to shape the behavior by looking for and rewarding behaviors that were just a little closer to the end result I wanted. My trainer helped me figure out what incremental steps to reward: look at the teeter, approach it, sniff it, touch it with her nose, touch it with her paw, put one paw on it, put two paws on it, stand on it with four paws, walk one step on it, walk several steps, walk to where it tips, tip it, walk the whole length of the board, trot the whole thing. We moved at Blue's pace; some sessions she might learn three new incremental steps; sometimes she might not try anything new.

I never "corrected" her; there was no "bad" behavior, just behaviors that were rewarded and behaviors that were ignored. Because I wasn't luring Blue or showing her what to do, she had to discover how to learn. I could see the wheels turning in her head; she was eager to figure out what movement was going to earn the click, praise and treat. She wanted to learn, and not just for the treats. Because the brain releases dopamine when mammals learn something new, it literally feels good to learn. Dogs who have

opportunities to discover what pleases their people love training
and love to learn.

It took months, but Blue learned to navigate the teeter-totter
like a pro. She did it because learning how to do it was fun and
interesting (in other words, intrinsically rewarding), not because I
demanded it of her or even because I gave her treats to do it (in
other words, extrinsically rewarding). Now nine years old, Blue
performs the teeter flawlessly in agility classes and trials.

But consider how enthusiastic and confident any dog would be
about approaching a wobbly, tipping board if we expected him to
perform like an adult when he was just a puppy. Or if the training
had been negative, demanding, critical and required instant per-
fection. Yet that's how we often treat ourselves.

You can shape your own writing behavior by giving yourself
frequent small rewards for incremental steps along the way to a
larger goal. Expecting "adult performance" from a writer or a
project that's still in the "puppy" stage is doomed to fail.

Shape-shifting

I know people are more complicated than dogs, but it really is
possible to shape your own behavior. When my friend Julie Theobald joined The Marsh, an upscale health club in a suburb of
Minneapolis, several months went by without her actually going
to the club. Julie realized that if she was paying so much for dues,
she might as well go. She started by telling herself that all she had
to do was drive to The Marsh. After she drove there and then

drove home a couple of times, Julie thought, "Well, since I'm driving there, I might as well go in." So she drove to The Marsh, parked her car, went inside and then went home again. After a while Julie thought, "Well, since I'm inside, I might as well check out the locker room." Then it was several days of, "Well, since I'm in the locker room, I might as well put on my swimsuit." This was followed by a week or so of, "Well, since I have my suit on, I may as well sit in the hot tub for a few minutes." After a several visits of, "Since I have my swimsuit on and I'm warmed up from the hot tub, I might as well get in the pool for five minutes and see what the water aerobics class is like," Julie stayed in class longer and longer. Eventually she acquired a sustainable habit of working out for an hour and a half several times a week.

If Julie had thought, "I'm paying all this money; I'd better get my lazy butt off the couch and get over to The Marsh and work out for two hours," she probably would have just canceled her membership. Instead, she shaped her behavior by rewarding herself (with positive self-talk and a sense of accomplishment) and slowly upping the ante just a little bit.

Eileen Peterson shaped her writing behavior with a four-step method posted on her office wall:

1. Show up in office.
2. Turn on computer.
3. Open writing file.
4. Write one sentence.

Eileen gives herself a small reward for completing each of these four steps. Most days, those four steps are all it takes to get her started writing. Eileen rewards herself for the routine, mechanical steps to get her past the initial inertia; then the intrinsic motivation takes over and she's on her way.

CHALLENGE: TRAINING SCHEDULE

Julie Theobald had an intuitive knack for upping the ante just right; she didn't make the next challenge so big or go to the next step so fast that she wanted to quit, and she didn't stop challenging herself until she'd reached her ultimate goal. You can try shaping your writing behavior by the seat of your pants, but I found in training Blue and in training myself that it really helps to know in advance what incremental steps I'm looking for and what rewards I'm going to give.

I encourage you to set up a "training schedule" for your writing that breaks a project into incremental stages and clarifies what "approximate behaviors" you want to recognize and reward. Identify in advance what small rewards you'll give yourself for daily actions (like showing up and putting in Product Time), what medium rewards you'll get for intermediate stages (like completing a chapter), and what large rewards you earn for major accomplishments (like completing a draft or revision of an entire manuscript).

INSIDE THE WRITER'S BRAIN: MIX 'EM UP

Research by Dr. Wolfram Schultz shows that unpredictable rewards are three to four times more exciting to dopamine neurons than predictable rewards.[117]

It's physically impossible to surprise yourself enough to, say, tickle yourself, but you can apply random numbers to help you surprise yourself with rewards. Create a numbered list of twenty-five small rewards, twenty-five medium rewards, and twenty-five large rewards in advance. After you've put in your time or achieved a milestone, decide what size reward is appropriate for your effort. Then pick a number out of a hat or use a random generator for the numbers 1 through 25 (you can find random number generators on the Internet) to select the specific reward you get.

Not only does this keep these rewards from becoming contingent, if-then rewards, it allows you to benefit from exciting dopamine neurons in your anterior cingulate in anticipation of a reward and still get maximum excitement from keeping the rewards mysterious.

Because studies show that altruism activates the reward centers of the brain and that, for some people, giving to others is more rewarding than receiving cash rewards themselves, it makes brain sense to include donations to your favorite charities and causes in your lists of twenty-five rewards.[18]

INQUIRY

"What was the best reward I ever received? What made that so special? How could I replicate that in my writing?"

8

WHY IS IT SO HARD TO WRITE, REVISITED

Anti-success Story

For some writers, it's a whisper of self-doubt: "You're probably not good enough," or, "What if you just don't have what it takes?" or, "Who's going to want to read what I write? Maybe I should just give up."

For some writers, it's a roar of criticism and abuse: "That's a stupid way to start a sentence," or, "This will never make sense," or, "This is boring, melodramatic, awkward, too far out there," or, "I must be stupid to even try to get my writing into the world."

For some writers, it's false advice that promises shelter, but delivers stagnation: "This piece isn't ready to go out; hold on to it for a while," or, "There's no point in entering that contest or applying for a grant; I won't win anyway," or, "Save yourself the pain of rejection."

For some writers, it's a collection of excuses and reasons to delay: "There's not enough time today," or, "I'm not inspired," or, "I need to pick up the kids, stop at the store, do the laundry and the cleaning, and walk the dog first."

For some writers, it's less-than-conscious beliefs and behaviors that make it harder to write: losing computer files, getting minor injuries and illnesses, cluttering your work space with other distractions, picking a fight with your partner, or picking one person after another who isn't worthy of being in a relationship with you.

For some writers, it's self-destructive behaviors that range from occasional overindulgence that leaves them too tired, bloated or hungover to write the next day, to full-fledged addictions: Raymond Chandler, Dorothy Parker, Jack Kerouac and Stephen King are just a few writers noted for being alcoholics/drug addicts or recovering alcoholics/drug addicts.

"It" is the Saboteur, and it's determined to make writing as difficult as possible for every writer. But it is not undefeatable—you can learn strategies to fight the Saboteur. And it's not all bad news—if you weren't creative, the Saboteur wouldn't bother to fight you. By the end of this chapter, you will have reasons and ways to celebrate the fact that you're lucky—and smart—enough to face the Saboteur's challenges.

The Saboteur May or May Not Be Your Inner Critic

Don't mistake the Inner Critic for the Saboteur. Although the Inner Critic can be a painful part of the Saboteur, it's not the only part or even the most significant aspect of this dangerous arche-type. And the Inner Critic is not necessarily the Saboteur. We must distinguish between two types of Inner Critic: the discerning critic and the damaging critic, a.k.a. the Saboteur.

The discerning critic accepts the writing as it is and appreciates what it can be. This acceptance allows a discerning writer to evaluate her or his work honestly and make effective changes. Discernment without judgment reveals possibilities that allow you to improve the current work and to develop the craft skills to keep growing as a writer. The damaging critic, on the other hand, makes preliminary judgments and sweeping generalizations that completely and irrevocably damn the writing and the writer without ever truly seeing and understanding the writing and its potential.

Judgment never serves a writer. Judgment poisons your ability to discern what's working in your writing and what you can do to improve it. Judgment precludes possibilities. Judgment is the tool of the Saboteur.

Psychological Origins of the Saboteur

Everyone has a Saboteur. According to Caroline Myss, author of *Sacred Contracts*, the Saboteur is one of the four powerful archetypes that are present in all of us. Myss says the Saboteur "reflects your fears of taking responsibility for yourself and what you create."[1]

Although some psychotherapists, like Francis Welter,[2] suggest the Saboteur (what he calls the Predator Archetype) serves the purpose of challenging us to transform, in my years of teaching and coaching, I've found nothing redeeming in the Saboteur itself. The Saboteur is a part of us that takes perverse delight in torturing us and engaging in self-destruction. It is a warped piece of another archetype that does have a purpose: the Inner Destroyer.

In *Dancing in the Dragon's Den*, I discuss how creation and destruction are opposite ends of the same pendulum. They are the poles of the life-force continuum. You cannot create without destroying. As Pablo Picasso says, "Every act of creation is first of all an act of destruction."

All of us express both the Creator archetype and the Destroyer archetype. We are both creative and destructive. Yet our Western tradition polarizes creativity as good and destruction as bad, despite the fact that this isn't necessarily so.

It is possible—and more than possible, necessary—to find healthy, life-affirming ways to express destructive energy. I've learned the hard way that if I want a good crop of carrots, I have to actually destroy the majority of the carrot seeds that sprout. And if I want good writing, I have to sprout lots of ideas and images, transplant them into sentences, and then prune many of those sentences.

But we are enculturated to the idea that destruction is wrong. As long as we believe destruction is bad, we put destruction in the shadow, which Carl Jung defined as "the person we have no wish to be," in other words, the traits, beliefs and behaviors we deny are part of us. We try to ignore the destructive energy that runs through us, that runs through all living creatures. Instead of finding healthy ways to consciously release destructive energy, we repress it, so it comes out sideways in unhealthy, unconscious ways. We break something. We get sick or injure ourselves. We are hypercritical of our creativity, ourselves or others. We have accidents. We engage in addictions or other forms of self-destruction.

When we deny our capacity for destruction, we limit our capacity for creativity. We also create and feed the Saboteur.

Carl Jung said the shadow is 90 percent gold. In other words, the vast majority of what we've put into the shadow and try to ignore and repress is actually treasure. It's not nearly as bad as we fear. It is our creative and spiritual potential. It is the fullness of our humanity that will allow us to feel compassion for ourselves and others if only we can find a way to acknowledge our shadow.

The Saboteur is part of that other 10 percent that is apparently beyond redemption. When we deny our capacity for destruction and push it into the shadow, it turns and twists back on us. An appropriate urge to destroy that is part of the cycle becomes self-destruction in ways that are not healthy or life-affirming. Disowned and disrespected, part of the Destroyer becomes the Saboteur.

INSIDE THE WRITER'S BRAIN: PHYSIOLOGICAL ORIGINS OF THE SABOTEUR

In *My Stroke of Insight*, brain scientist and stroke survivor Dr. Jill Bolte Taylor writes, "I whole-heartedly believe that 99.999 percent of the cells in my brain and body want me to happy, healthy and successful. A tiny portion of the story-teller [part of the brain], however, does not seem to be unconditionally attached to my joy, and is excellent at exploring thought patterns that have the potential to really derail my feeling of inner peace."[3]

Taylor theorizes that a collection of neurons in the language centers of the left hemisphere is the origin of negative thought patterns and negative emotions of jealousy, fear and rage. This sounds very much like the self-destructive behaviors that arise from what I call the Saboteur. Taylor suggests that the "negative story-teller" is at most the size of a peanut and observes that it was a relief when this part of her brain was silenced by the stroke.[4]

But as Taylor points out, recovering from her stroke meant the Peanut Gallery, as she calls this peanut-size patch of cranky neurons, started to natter and nag again. Aware of the Peanut Gallery's propensity for negativity, Taylor gives permission for this part of her to whine only at specified and limited times during the day. Persistently noticing what thoughts she's entertaining keeps the Peanut Gallery in check.

"Having said that, however," Taylor acknowledges, "I am often humored by the scheming antics of my story-teller in response to this type of directive. I have found that just like little children, these cells may challenge the authority of my authentic voice and test my conviction. Once asked to be silent, they tend to pause for a moment and then immediately reengage those forbidden loops."[5]

If Taylor's conscious focus falters, "those uninvited loops can generate new strength and begin monopolizing my mind again . . . I have also found that when I am least expecting it—feeling either physically tired or emotionally vulnerable—those negative circuits have a tendency to raise their hurtful heads."[6]

Success Story

Even though author Jacquelyn B. Fletcher has known about the concept of the Saboteur since college, and learned to recognize and respond to variations on the "You're not good enough" theme her Saboteur prefers, and has even written about the Inner Critic for *Writer's Digest* (November 2005), she can still be surprised by her Saboteur.

Laughing gently, she says, "It absolutely helps to know about the Saboteur, but it's still a surprise when I discover, 'Oh, I've totally sabotaged myself again.' I used to believe it when my Saboteur said I wasn't good enough. I sent work out too quickly and I couldn't stand up when I got feedback. I tried to please everybody and ended up destroying a couple of pieces because I wasn't confident enough in my own abilities."

As Jacque learned to respond to her Saboteur more effectively, how she saw that part of herself changed. "It used to be Gollum from *The Lord of the Rings*. I got a Gollum action figure at Target and when it said, 'My precious,' in its creepy voice, I'd get chills, but I'd laugh at myself and keep writing. But then it became something that was even more terrifying—it looked a lot more like me and said, 'You're not good enough.' It was me saying that to myself, in a strange way. And because it was more like me, it was harder to get around. It seemed like it was telling me the truth."

Jacque has shifted from the old, adversarial relationship she once had with her Saboteur. "Now it's this little monkey, something I should have compassion for as a creature who is not as evolved. It was a spiritual evolution. When I'm aware of my Higher Power in my meditations, I can see that I'm really just this human wrapping around the Divine inside of me. So I have more compassion for the human part of me because it's just doing the best it can."

Meditation is a big part of how Jacque keeps her Saboteur in check. "I think the novel I just finished is one of the most mature pieces I've ever done. I finished it by doing meditations around, 'Okay, monkey mind, shhhh.' Treating that part of me like a little baby was how I could bring my writing to that new level."

Jacque has also designed her own "PhD program" in children's literature (to follow the MFA she earned at Emerson College in Boston). Reading dozens of children's books every week highlighted that her Saboteur was lying when it said she wasn't good enough. It also increased her ability to discern where her writing was strong and where she can improve her craft.

Jacque advises, "It's vital that you develop ways to cope with the Saboteur. If you don't, the Saboteur will push you away from your writing for your whole life, and you'll end up on your deathbed without doing what you intend to do. We have these skills and talents for a reason, and that reason is bigger than our insecurities and fears."

Know Your Enemy

As Jacque Fletcher pointed out, the Saboteur can and will morph. If you're to have any hope of responding effectively to the Saboteur, you need to recognize its many guises. Your Saboteur will be unique, but there are five major forms to watch for: the Attacker, the Enticer, the Protector, the Innocent, and the Unlucky.

When people think of the Saboteur, the Attacker is what usually comes to mind. This is the hypercritical voice that nags, threatens, insults, judges, denigrates and disparages you. But as painful as that is, the Saboteur can do worse: it can disguise itself with one of its softer, subtler faces so that you can't tell when you're being self-destructive and undermining your creativity.

The Enticer is the smiling face of the Saboteur that reassures you that everything is okay and your goals will be magically fulfilled without needing to face challenges or exert real effort. The Enticer deals in fantasy and lulls you into inaction.

The Attacker sucker punches you; the Enticer soothes. The Attacker rages and screams; the Enticer whispers in your head. The Attacker predicts rejection, disappointment and doom (based on your assumed failings as a writer); the Enticer promises a sweet tomorrow you don't even have to work for today.

This form of the Saboteur will sweetly sympathize, "You've had a really hard day. It won't matter if you:

- "Skip Process today."
- "Take the day off from writing."

- "Relax in front of the TV or with a computer game instead of going to the Y."
- "Have a cookie, just one, just one more . . . well, you may as well finish the bag now."
- "Wait until tomorrow; there's always tomorrow."

The wide-eyed Innocent form of the Saboteur watches in stunned surprise when creative endeavors don't go as planned. This voice will say with all apparent sincerity, "How could this happen to me?"

While the true innocence of recognizing what you don't know and asking open-ended questions is essential to the creative process, the Innocent face of the Saboteur is a calculated pretense. True innocence is open to growing through experience; the faux innocence of the Saboteur has no intention of changing or letting you get unstuck.

Maya Angelou says, "When you know better, you do better." The Innocent claims it doesn't have the information or experience to know anything for sure, and since it never knows better, it never lets you do better.

The Innocent deals in denial and inaction. Terminal indecisiveness makes it impossible to take action and move forward, therefore guaranteeing that your creative dreams will remain unfulfilled. And all the while, the Innocent will shrug and say:

- "I don't know what to do."
- "I can't figure this out."
- "Maybe I should wait until I'm not so confused."

- "I wish someone would help me."
- "It's not my fault; I didn't choose this."

The Protector form of the Saboteur promises to keep you safe from rejection, criticism and failure. Of course, it doesn't admit that this safety means isolating yourself and your writing so that you also remove yourself from opportunities to receive acceptance, encouragement, discerning observations that could help you improve the writing, and, ultimately, success.

While the Attacker disparages your ability to ever finish anything worthwhile and the Innocent pretends you don't know what to do, the Protector encourages you to keep tweaking, editing and rewriting. As long as the writing is a work in process, it can't be criticized or rejected.

The Protector sounds like it has your best interests at heart and croons like an overprotective mother:

- "There's no sense in rushing to rejection. Make sure you do everything you possibly can before submitting it."
- "It's too risky. Wait until you have a better shot at winning a contest."
- "Why set yourself up for failure? You know how awful it feels when someone doesn't like your writing."
- "Be careful who you show your writing to. Hang back and see what happens first. Oops, now it's too late. Well, maybe next time, dear."
- "Maybe I should take a break from keeping a journal until I feel more secure."

Sometimes sabotage comes in the form of accidents, injuries, illness, even relationships. Of course, sometimes an accident is just an accident; even Freud said sometimes a cigar is just a cigar. But when the term "accident-prone" comes to mind, when there's a repeating pattern behind the injuries, or when you end one unhealthy relationship just to get into another, consider the possibility that the Unlucky Saboteur is at work.

Please note that I am not making the New Agey assumption that if something bad happens in your life, you caused it. I don't think people get cancer, for example, because they "wanted to create that for themselves on some level." Misfortune is not a sign that you're sabotaging yourself. But your Saboteur can and will make the most of any misfortune to interfere with your writing. And it will emphasize how bad your bad luck is and ignore the positive side of any situation.

The Unlucky deals in disappointment and dejection. It will heave a huge sigh and say:

- "What's the point?"
- "Someone else has probably done it before."
- "Publishing is all about who you know, and I just don't have the connections."
- "Someone will steal my idea."
- "I just can't catch a break."

The Unlucky Saboteur is a real inner Eeyore, and listening to it will only make a sad gray ass out of you.

Five Faces, Four Characteristics, One Goal

You need to know these four key characteristics of the Saboteur.

The Saboteur Always Lies

Sometimes the Saboteur will tell outright, bald-faced whoppers, adopting Hitler's Big Lie approach—tell an outrageous lie loud enough and frequently enough and people will believe it. Often the Saboteur twists a partial truth to create a lie, for example, "Three magazines have rejected my piece (true), so it must be a bad idea (not necessarily true), and I'm a complete failure as a writer (lie)."

The Saboteur loves to draw false and hurtful conclusions from incomplete information. The Attacker and Unlucky Saboteurs exaggerate the negative aspect of any situation and dismiss any positives; the Innocent refuses to recognize truth; the Enticer uses fantasy and inflated positivity against you; and the Protector says, "I told you so. Better not try that again."

The Saboteur Is Never Satisfied

No matter how hard you try, no matter how much you accomplish, no matter how much good your friends and allies see in you, it will never be enough for the Saboteur. This is the unending litany of, "You're not good enough, smart enough, published enough, credentialed and degreed enough, recognized enough, persistent enough, witty enough, young enough (or old enough)." Unless, of course, you're too good, too smart, published too much in this genre, too credentialed and degreed (overqualified and out of touch), too famous, too persistent, too clever for your own good, and too young (or too old).

Whatever you do, it's not the right thing. You could spend hours every day for months making fabulous progress on a novel, and your Saboteur will say, "It's been months since you've even looked at your poetry. Oh, and your family hates you now." Whatever you are, it's not the right thing.

Sherri H., another writer in my writers' group, was afraid that her experience as a journalist would interfere with writing memoir, while I was concerned that without a journalism background I wouldn't be able to conduct the kind of interviews that made other brain books effective. The Saboteur wants us to see everything about ourselves as bugs and flaws—but the truth is, all these things are features and strengths. The real truth is that Sherri has strengths she gained as a journalist that she can legitimately claim in her grant application and leverage in her memoir. I'm not writing the kind of brain book other authors write, and I bring experiences—like my years of coaching—to this book that other authors couldn't.

The Saboteur Knows Where You Are Vulnerable and It Always Goes for the Throat

After all, your Saboteur is you, so of course it knows what will hurt the most. If you lean toward perfectionism, your Saboteur will point out each and every mistake you make, taking particular glee in those that have gone out into the world already so you can't easily correct them, and insist that if you can't do it perfectly, you shouldn't even try. If you have doubts about your credibility, your Saboteur will highlight other people's credentials, insist you really should get a more advanced degree, and constantly tell you that you're a fraud. The Saboteur will attack wherever you are most vulnerable and afraid.

The Saboteur Is Never Going to Go Away

It's like the Tar Baby in the B'rer Rabbit stories. The more you try to reason or argue with your Saboteur, the more entangled you get. Fighting the Saboteur is like playing a never-ending game of Whack-A-Mole—just when you think you've figured it out, the Saboteur will morph into a different form and use different techniques. You can't get rid of the Saboteur and you can't control it.

But you can learn to respond so that the Saboteur no longer controls you. Every time you respond appropriately, you reduce how much influence the Saboteur has. You can reduce how frequently and persistently it will show up, but you can never assume it's gone for good.

The Saboteur is at its nastiest when you take action to further your dreams. So you may be tempted to appease it by giving up on your creativity, hoping that if you don't rock the boat, the Saboteur will stop attacking you. And it might. Giving in to the Saboteur can provide temporary relief. As you block your creativity and lose awareness of who you really are and what you really want, the Saboteur usually gets quieter—for a while, anyway.

But the ultimate cost of trying to appease the Saboteur is diminished self-esteem, unfulfilled dreams and feeling spiritually disconnected and confused. Worst of all, the Saboteur never really goes away. It's only quiet for a while, and when it returns, it is stronger and more vicious, like a junkyard dog that's been rewarded by your timidity. You only wanted to get the Saboteur to stop criticizing you, but appeasing it has fed it. It's like a mythical monster that seems to get bigger and more powerful no matter what you do to fight it.

Vicious or seductive, innocent, protective, or unlucky, all forms of the Saboteur have one common purpose: to keep you from writing by making you miserable and destroying your self-confidence and self-esteem.

Don't Give In and Don't Give Up

Your Saboteur won't go away and it won't play nice. But you're not going away, you're not going to abandon your writing, and you don't have to play nice either.

You don't have to let the Saboteur run and ruin your life. Your best strategy is to observe your Saboteur closely. Notice which faces of the Saboteur are most active in your life.

Which forms show up most frequently? I see the Attacker and Enticer forms more than the Innocent, Protector or Unlucky. Learn to recognize your Saboteur's voice—is it nasty, seductive, baffled, condescending or whiny? Take note of the kinds of things each of Saboteur's five forms say. Highlight key phrases. Pay attention to the habits and behaviors your Saboteur uses to delay or inhibit your writing. Learn to recognize your Saboteur—the faster you recognize it, the less havoc it can wreck.

It can be a relief to recognize your Saboteur. After all, the Saboteur always lies, so when you recognize the voice of your Saboteur, you know what it says is simply untrue. Alerted to the Saboteur's presence, you're willing and able to take corrective action. One of the best ways to challenge the Saboteur is to refuse to accept its lies as truth.

Another effective strategy is to refuse to let your Saboteur call the shots. Ignore its demands. The Saboteur is never willing to be ignored, so it takes a bit of effort to keep telling yourself, "That's just my Saboteur; I don't have to pay attention." But it is possible, and it's liberating to know what's going on. When you remind yourself, "Oh, that's just my Saboteur," use the same neutral tone that you'd use to observe any other frequent but unimportant occurrence. Ignore its suggestions. Just keep doing what you set out to do.

Do not let the Saboteur detour you from honoring your commitments, no matter how sweetly—or viciously or bemusedly or patronizingly or despairingly—it talks to you.

Success Story

John Drozdal used to have "pretty much every excuse possible to avoid writing or, worse yet, to cast aspersions on my ability to even write at all. 'It's too late in the day; it's too early in the morning; I'm too tired; I need to clean, do the dishes, shower, make a pot of coffee, check the baseball scores, call my therapist, and run a marathon before I am ready to write' were common thoughts running through my head."

John named his Saboteur Sergei because it bears a striking resemblance to Boris Badenov, Rocky the Flying Squirrel's nemesis. "Boris's preoccupation was to 'give squirrel bad time,'" John recalls. "Sergei enjoys giving me an equally bad time about my writing."

Once John recognized that this was his Saboteur talking and that, as far as Sergei was concerned, there would never be any hope of writing today, tomorrow or ever, John was determined to change the old delaying tactics.

"When I sense Sergei is paying a visit, I simply greet him before he does his mischief. I say, 'Hello, Sergei. I'm much too busy writing and don't have time for your interruptions, so kiss off.' It usually works, and he goes back to his underground abode."

John is done with excuses—Sergei still suggests them of course, but John's not buying. "The biggest accomplishment I gained from facing my Saboteur is the ability to keep consistently showing up for my writing commitments. I'm convinced every writer and creative person has a Saboteur. I encourage other writers to get acquainted with their Saboteurs, learn their behaviors and how to head them off at the pass."

CHALLENGES: RECOGNIZE THE SABOTEUR

As John Drozdal suggests, you need to know your Saboteur when it shows up. The following short exercises will lead you through some detective work to clarify what your Saboteur looks, sounds and acts like, so you can recognize it faster the next time it tries to sneak up on you.

Freewrite

Quickly complete the following sentences. These are all very metaphoric, so there is no one right way to respond or even a "logical" response. Just jot down your first thoughts.

If my Saboteur had a color, it would be:
If my Saboteur had a shape, it would be:
If my Saboteur had a texture, it would be:
If my Saboteur had a sound, it would be:
If my Saboteur had a smell, it would be:
If my Saboteur had a name, it would be:
If my Saboteur were an animal, it would be:
If my Saboteur were a natural disaster, it would be:
If my Saboteur were a fictional character, it would be:

Draw the Saboteur's Mug Shot

Your next detective task is to draw your Saboteur. You don't have to know what your Saboteur looks like before you start drawing, although you might have a pretty good idea by now. Sometimes the process of drawing reveals new information. Don't worry about your drawing skills; it's not as if you should care what your Saboteur thinks about the drawing anyway. And since the Saboteur is never satisfied, it won't like the drawing no matter what you do. Play with color and shape and see what happens.

Brainstorm the Rap Sheet Possibilities

Your next detecting task is to prepare your Saboteur's rap sheet. Start by brainstorming potential crimes your Saboteur may have committed.

- Murdered hope
- Assaulted my self-esteem
- Pillaged my creative energy
- Slandered, robbed, committed hit-and-run, battery, grand theft novel, fraud . . .

Now that you have some possibilities to get you started, write your Saboteur's rap sheet. What specific crimes has your Saboteur committed? Consider the harm done to you, to your creativity and to your community. By undermining you, perhaps your Saboteur has delayed the completion of a novel or chapbook or collection of essays that could benefit your future readers more than you know.

Write the Eviction Notice

Write a letter informing your Saboteur that it is no longer welcome and you're not going to let it push you around anymore.

Respond to the Saboteur

You might think that with all these detective metaphors, I'm going to recommend you get your inner detective hot on the case and that you spend a lot of energy chasing the Saboteur like a crime-fighting superhero, arrest it, put it on trial and lock it away. But I don't recommend channeling too much energy into pursuing the Saboteur.

What you need is a way to keep the Saboteur at a safe distance. In "Squelch Your Inner Censor" Jacque Fletcher writes, "A friend thinks of her censor as a prissy Barbie doll. She bought a doll, and every time she gets stuck with the critic, she drops the doll into her metal trash can, which slams shut with a very satisfying sound. Then she continues to write."[7]

Having a simple, quick ritual like this to remind yourself not to engage with your Saboteur can be effective and satisfying. Don't try to put the Saboteur on trial; you'll only get caught in a quagmire of arguing with it. Remember the fourth characteristic of the Saboteur: it's never going to go away. The more you try to fight the Saboteur, the more powerful it becomes. Just notice it—"Oh, there's my Saboteur again"—drop it in a trash can if you want, and keep doing what you set out to do.

Destroy the Saboteur

Remember, it is our reluctance to express destructive energy that feeds the Saboteur, so it's very effective to release destruction energy on the Saboteur. It's also very satisfying. Tear up the pages with the Saboteur's description and rap sheet. Shred its mug shot. Stomp on the pieces if you want. Some people get a kick out of making a model of the Saboteur out of clay or Play-Doh and then smashing it.

An Obsession of a Different Color

An innovative therapy for obsessive-compulsive disorder (OCD) trains patients to acknowledge their obsessive thoughts as no more than faulty brain signals that they do not need to act on. Can we do the same with the Saboteur? Can writers learn to recognize saboteur thinking as faulty signals arising from unconscious self-destructive impulses and refuse to believe the thoughts or act on them?

Dr. Norman Doidge, author of *The Brain That Changes Itself*, seems to think so. He declares that the plasticity-based OCD treatment developed by UCLA psychiatrist Jeffrey M. Schwartz can "help not only those with obsessive-compulsive disorder but also those of us with more everyday worries, when we start stewing about something and can't stop even though we know it's pointless . . . or when we become compulsive and driven by such 'nasty habits' as compulsive nail biting, hair pulling, shopping, gambling and eating. Even some forms of obsessive jealousy, substance abuse, compulsive sexual behaviors and excessive concern about what others think about us, self-image, the body and self-esteem can be helped."[8]

My experience and that of my clients and students has convinced me that Schwartz's approach can be effectively applied to resolving obsessive thinking (about what we have to do before we can write or how fatally flawed our writing is and so on), obsessive self-criticism, self-doubt and risk avoidance—in other words, the Saboteur.

In *The Mind and the Brain*, Schwartz writes, "One of the most striking aspects of OCD urges is that, except in the most severe cases, they are what is called ego-dystonic: they seem apart from, and at odds with, one's intrinsic sense of self. They seem to arise from a part of the mind that is not you, as if a hijacker were taking over your brain's controls. . . . Patients with obsessive-compulsive disorder experience an urge to wash their hands, for instance, while fully cognizant of the fact that their hands are not dirty."[9]

Self-destructive impulses from the Saboteur are typically ego-dystonic as well. For example, many writers know intellectually that their best strategy is to complete a draft no matter how "shitty" (as Anne Lamott would say) it is. But they can't fight the urge to rewrite the first pages over and over, in the same way OCD patients can't, for example, fight the urge to wash their hands over and over even though they know their hands are clean. When we're in the grip of the Saboteur, like when a patient is in the grip of OCD, there is a split between what we know ("I should finish the draft," or "I know my hands are clean") and what we feel ("But I have to rewrite this one little bit," or "But I have to wash one more time").

Let's be clear: OCD is not the Saboteur, and experiencing saboteur thinking does not mean you have OCD. OCD is a clearly defined "neuropsychiatric disease"[10] that is caused by dysfunction in three distinct areas of the brain. The Saboteur, meanwhile, is a theory and a psychological concept. I know of no systematic research investigating the Saboteur; all evidence is anecdotal. But even though OCD is a far more devastating disorder than the typical writer's struggles with the Saboteur, we can still draw some useful parallels and apply Schwartz's success in treating OCD to our efforts to muzzle the Saboteur.

INSIDE THE WRITER'S BRAIN:
WHEN SOMETHING GOES WRONG

The orbital frontal cortex is the brain's error detector. When something unexpected happens, this region of the cortex just behind our eyes starts firing, sending signals that something is wrong to the cingulate gyrus, which lies deeper in the cortex.[11]

A normally functioning orbital frontal cortex is probably part of what alerts us to something unexpected or "off" in our writing. A discerning writer not in the grips of saboteur thinking recognizes messages from the orbital frontal cortex without judgment and asks open-ended questions like, "What specifically is 'off' in this section? Why is this piece of writing not working? How can I make it better?"

Brain scans show that in OCD, the orbital frontal cortex is hyperactive and keeps sending the "something is wrong" message to the cingulate gyrus. Although the Saboteur probably doesn't interfere with the orbital frontal cortex's normal functioning, it is like OCD in the way it tends to inflate, exaggerate and repeat warnings from the orbital frontal cortex. It also adds its own warped interpretation that the writing and the writer are fatally flawed and there is no hope of improvement.

When the cingulate gyrus receives the "something is wrong" message, it sends signals to the heart and gut, creating both the mental and physiological feelings of anxiety and dread that moti-

vate us to take action. A discerning writer not crippled by the Saboteur recognizes this uneasiness as a sign that corrective action is
needed and experiments with different ways to improve the writing and fix what's "off."

But a writer in the clutches of the Saboteur, like an OCD
patient with a hyperactive cingulate gyrus, experiences heightened
feelings of anxiety, dread or hopelessness. It may well be that
thinking saboteur thoughts ("This sucks. I'll never figure this out.
Why did I ever think I could write? I'm going to fail") increases
activity in the cingulate gyrus.

People with OCD are driven by intense feelings of dread (triggered by the hyperactive cingulate gyrus) to repeat compulsive
behaviors (to wash their hands, count their steps, check and recheck
that the stove is turned off) that they know intellectually won't
solve the problem, in a futile attempt to ease the anxiety. Likewise,
a writer wrapped up in saboteur thinking seems to lose the ability
to take reasonable corrective action. Instead, she/he engages in
self-defeating behaviors and does little or nothing to improve the
current writing, situation and her/his mastery of the craft.

In a normal brain, when the caudate nucleus (a part of the limbic system that serves as a kind of switching station for the signals
it receives from many other regions of the brain) recognizes that
we've taken action to correct the error, it signals the orbital frontal
cortex and cingulate gyrus to stop firing.

A discerning writer will recognize the "all is well" signal from
the caudate nucleus with awareness that nothing is ever perfect
but that she/he has done what she/he can with the writing, that
good enough is good enough, and move on. But like an OCD

patient with a "sticky" caudate nucleus that can't shift gears, a writer immersed in saboteur thinking will deny the "all is well" signal. Nothing is ever good enough for the Saboteur.

INSIDE THE WRITER'S BRAIN: ERASING OCD

As Hebb's Law ("neurons that fire together, wire together") predicts, the more an OCD patient focuses on the content of the disorder (germs, the possibility that the door is unlocked, etc.) and practices the compulsion (washing hands, checking the door), the worse the disorder becomes. Doidge observes, "OCD often worsens with time, gradually altering the structure of the brain . . . with OCD, worry begets worry."[12]

It is reasonable to assume that prolonged saboteur thinking, like prolonged, regular mediation practice or other mental habits, can eventually influence how the brain functions. And as Hebb's Law suggests, we can reverse those negative effects by changing how we think.

Applying some principles of the Buddhist meditation he practices, Schwartz teaches patients to mindfully observe the universal form of OCD without focusing on the specific content of their own obsessions and compulsions. Schwartz's treatment directs patients to "relabel" and "reattribute" their experience. They are not being attacked by germs, for example; they are experiencing false thoughts (relabeling what is happening) that are caused by pathological brain dysfunctions and therefore are not part of the patient's true self (reattributing why it's happening).[13]

In the same way, learning to recognize the Saboteur allows writers to relabel and reattribute the negative thoughts. They are not bad writers who are incapable of improvement and need to be careful to avoid rejection, for example; they are hearing the lies of the Saboteur's inner monologue. They need not follow the warped thinking of the Saboteur, but can simply dismiss those misleading thoughts and continue with the writing or other activity they originally planned.

Schwartz knows this is not as easy as it might sound. But the payoff of such mindful effort is life changing. "Once I learned to identify my OCD symptoms as OCD rather than as 'important' content-laden thoughts that had to be deciphered for their deep meaning," one of Schwartz's patients reported, "I was partially freed from OCD."[14]

My coaching clients and students have made the same observation about the significance of recognizing that the Saboteur is alien to who they really are. This is why it's so effective to name your Saboteur, picture it as something that has a shape, texture and color, or think of it as an animal, natural disaster or fictional character. All of those are ways to remind yourself that your Saboteur is not who you really are.

Get Clear

The Saboteur thrives in uncertainty and ambiguity; intention and integrity are key to keeping it at bay. I cannot encourage you too strongly to make your commitments crystal clear. One of the reasons I recommend making a commitment to do Process, Self-care and Product Time for a predetermined amount of time is so you'll know when you can stop without letting the Saboteur have its way.

Know exactly what you are committing yourself to: what will you do, when will you start, how long will you do it, how many times, and what does and does not qualify as honoring your commitment? For example, "I will color for fifteen minutes starting at eight p.m. five times this week. If I prefer, drawing or sewing are acceptable substitutions." You can change your mind, of course, deciding that you're going to color in the afternoon instead, for example, but do not deviate from the plan once you've started coloring or the start time has arrived. Thinking, "Maybe I'll just do ten minutes tonight," invites the Saboteur in.

WRITER'S APPLICATION: CHOOSE YOUR RESPONSE

Like John Drozdal, you can learn to recognize when your Sergei is making an appearance. Like Jill Bolte Taylor, you can recognize that the saboteur thoughts arise from nothing more than a peanut-size collection of neurons that will tell the most outrageous whoppers to make you miserable, and you therefore refuse to entertain those thoughts. Like Jacque Fletcher, you can practice meditation and choose to feel compassion for the Saboteur as long as you don't let it push you away from your writing.

You can choose to respond to your Saboteur in any way that empowers you to dismiss its cruel, subtle, persistent lies and challenges. The more you refuse to let your Saboteur control you, the more you weaken that neural pathway and the less power the Saboteur has over you. You can, like Schwartz's patients, free yourself by changing how your brain works.

Remember, if you weren't expressing creative energy, you wouldn't generate the equal and opposite destructive energy that feeds the Saboteur. Find suitable ways to consciously dissipate that destructive energy (shred paper, break glass, smash what you make out of clay for Process play, etc.) so that it stops fueling the Saboteur.

You are now armed with the most important tool you need to effectively respond to the Saboteur—information. Be mindful and use it well.

INQUIRY

Fill in the blank in the following sentence to describe the kind of writer you are (e.g., "aspiring writer" or "emerging novelist"):

"If I were a spy given the job of sabotaging an _____ to ensure that that writer couldn't write, what would I do?"

After you answer this question, consider: "What can I do to prevent my Saboteur from doing this to me?"

9

FOUR STEPS TO RESOLVING RESISTANCE

Learning Story

When I was twenty-seven, I experienced the physically paralyzing power of resistance. Not in my writing—on the face of a cliff.

Going through a divorce I didn't want, I avoided the emptiness of our house on weekends by traveling to state parks to camp with my dog. On this particular day, a group of ten or twelve college kids were jumping off a cliff into the lake where I was swimming. It was a safe place to do this—the cliff was undercut so they couldn't possibly hit anything on the way down, and the lake was at least twenty feet deep, with no submerged rocks.

One young woman didn't want to jump, which wasn't unreasonable, since it looked like a twenty-five-foot leap. As her friends teased her good-naturedly, I got drawn into their banter. She admitted she was scared, and I tried to encourage her. When one of the other students asked me why I hadn't jumped yet, the fact that I was at least six years older than they never made me pause. I was a native of Wisconsin; these were college kids up from the Chicago area, so there was the "I can't let them show me up" thing. Besides, I was "outdoorsy"—I graduated Outward Bound, climbed mountains, and canoed whitewater rivers. Of course I could jump off this cliff.

But when I got to the top of the cliff, it was a lot higher when I was up there looking down than it had been when I was in the lake looking up.

I inched to the very edge. I shivered when I glanced down. I bent my knees and swung my arms to rock back and forward on my toes.

Swing. "One . . ."

Swing again. "Two . . ."

And swing one more time. "Three!"

I fully expected to jump on three. But my feet didn't move. I was frozen from the knees down and completely shocked that I still stood there.

"Okay," I said, as if I were talking to the college kids gathered around waiting for their turn. "On three."

Swing. "One . . ."

Swing again. "Two . . ."

Swing one last time. "Three!"

I didn't move.

It wasn't that I was having a debate with myself about whether I was going to jump or not. I fully intended to jump. I told myself to jump. But I was paralyzed.

My cortex planned to jump. My ego was fully committed to

jumping. I wanted to jump; I almost needed to jump to maintain my sense of identity. But my limbic system overrode that conscious intention and I didn't move.

You may recall that the limbic system doesn't have access to the language centers (which reside in the cortex), so my emotional brain didn't say anything. But if it could talk, it might have said something along the lines of, "No-no-no-no-no! Are you crazy? That's at least thirty feet down. You'll get us killed! I'm putting my foot down. In fact, I'm putting both feet down. I am *not* jumping off this cliff."

My limbic system wouldn't let my body do what my cortex wanted to do. If I had been smart, I would've listened to my limbic system and joined the young woman in enduring the embarrassing but harmless teasing of her friends. But I was stubborn and I wasn't going to let my fear control me this way.

My limbic system did let my legs move backward, and I walked away. I sat on a rock, took some deep breaths, and talked myself through my fear. "This is safe. They've all done it several times. This is just like the high dive at the pool, except it's twice as high. All I have to do is jump and remember to inhale as soon as my feet hit the water. I can do this. I'm doing this and everything is going to be all right."

It is possible to act in the face of our fears; otherwise none of us would ever do anything courageous and adventurous. It is possible to calm the body and reengage the cortex to move through resistance.

I went back to the edge of the cliff. I took a deep breath and jumped. I screamed, of course. Just before I jumped, I remembered the scene in *Butch Cassidy and the Sundance Kid* where Robert Redford and Paul Newman jump off the cliff, each of them holding one end of a gun belt, windmilling his other arm and yelling, "Ohhhhh, shiiiiiiiiit!" So I screamed, "Ohhhhh, shiiiiiiiiit!"

I realized I'd run out of breath and I still hadn't hit the water yet.

That flipped my limbic system back on and my cortex off. I should have listened to my limbic system the first time it kicked in, but this second time, plummeting off the cliff, was not a good time to lose my cortex's ability to anticipate future outcomes. For some insane reason—probably some misplaced instinct—I tried to climb back up, even though there was nothing to grab. I kicked my feet and windmilled my arms faster. This did keep my feet from hitting the water for a fraction of a second. In that fraction of a second of complete disregard for the consequences of this instinctual flailing around, my butt hit the water first. I made one of the most spectacular cannonball entries ever. I bruised my tailbone so badly, I had to spend the next week sitting on one of those inflatable doughnuts designed for hemorrhoid sufferers.

Looking back, it's a funny story and a great illustration of the power of resistance and the dilemma of figuring out which part of the brain to listen to. And I did learn valuable lessons. I experienced firsthand how profoundly paralyzing resistance can be. I proved to myself that I can override my resistance with willpower, that my cortex can reassert itself after a limbic system takeover. I also demonstrated—and felt the uncomfortable evidence of that demonstration—that it's not always wise to do so. And that once you are committed to the cortex's plan, it's probably best to do everything you can to keep that part of your brain in command for the duration of that plan.

What Went Wrong

So what went wrong? Why did this example of working through fear and overcoming resistance have such a painful outcome? By sharing this story, am I reversing my position, to suggest that maybe we should let our resistance and fear dictate what we do?

We can and should overcome our resistance, but we need to exercise care when we do. I used three out of four of the steps needed to resolve resistance effectively:

1. Recognize
2. Relax
3. Respect
4. Redirect

Missing that one step—respect—meant the difference between "effective" and "painful."

I did recognize my resistance. It was pretty hard to miss when my legs froze and I couldn't jump. I did take the time to breathe deeply and reassure myself so that I could relax and bring my cortex back online. And I did redirect the energy of the resistance into forward motion right off that cliff. But I didn't respect my resistance, which is why it resurfaced at the worst possible moment.

STEP ONE:
RECOGNIZE THE RESISTANCE

Resistance by Any Other Name

It's crucial that writers learn to call resistance by its correct name. Our verbal ability encourages us to think of a multitude of synonyms, and we think we're not writing because we're too busy, distracted, lazy, stupid, perfectionistic, unskilled or because we lack willpower and procrastinate too much. We forget that all of these are variations of writing resistance.

The challenge arises because the limbic system doesn't have language, so we don't have words for what we feel at times. The limbic system lacks the sophisticated thinking and nuanced analysis needed to recognize the subtler forms of resistance. Even a brain in the midst of a full-fledged limbic system takeover can recognize full-fledged writer's block, with its accompanying aphasia and paralysis, but this paralysis of wanting and needing to write and not being able to eke out the words is actually pretty rare. In fact, I suspect most writers either procrastinate or distract ourselves away from our writing to keep ourselves unaware that we do not or cannot write the way we want to. We're intelligent human beings; why wouldn't we do what we can to avoid that painful awareness? Fear makes us want to look away, but as the Japanese film director Akira Kurosawa said, "To be an artist means never to avert your eyes." We have to learn to see resistance for what it is, no matter what form it appears in.

Most forms of writer's resistance are subtler than full-fledged writer's block and therefore more difficult to recognize. Like the saying about alcoholics, recognizing you have a problem is always the most important step, because until you recognize you have a problem, you don't think about solving the problem.

There are probably as many unique ways to resist writing as there are writers, but resistance tends to fall into these forms:

Writer's Block
Full-fledged aphasia and paralysis, actually sitting down with the intention and desire to write and being unable to do so no matter how long you sit there and what you try.

Procrastination
Continually putting off the writing, thinking, "I should be writing and I will, but not right now," waiting until the last minute to get started, making the mistaken assumptions that you write better under pressure, that it will be easier later, or that you need more time than you have right now, so you shouldn't even start.

Postponing
Believing that some milestone must be passed before you can even consider writing, telling yourself you'll write in a few weeks, months or years after you (select one or several of the following): get a degree or other credential, quit your current job, find a new job, retire, get through the holidays, go on vacation, return from vacation, etc.

Distraction

Shifting focus from writing to one or several distractions, including electronic distractions (checking email, voice mail, IM, blogs, Twitter, Facebook or other social media, watching TV or DVDs, Internet shopping and surfing) office or household distractions (deciding to write just as soon as you finish some other task, like cleaning, organizing, laundry, filing, updating records, sorting the mail, looking for answers in the refrigerator, and sorting your sock drawer), personal and social distractions (recreational reading that gets out of hand, doing just one more crossword or sudoku puzzle, satisfying everyone else's needs at the expense of your own, needing to take care of another person or animal 24/7 even when that person or animal doesn't need you to do that).

Perfectionism

Setting unrealistically high demands, obsessively rewriting one section over and over, refusing to accept the necessity of moving forward with an imperfect draft, applying all-or-nothing thinking about the writing and your process ("If I can't get perfect conditions, there's no point in even trying to write"), being unwilling to trust the process and ignoring the reality that all ideas go through awkward stages before they're fully developed.

Hypercriticism and Excessive Pessimism

Related to perfectionism, hypercriticism and excessive pessimism go from all-or-nothing thinking to nothing-or-nothing thinking: assuming that everything you write is and always will be fatally flawed; seeing only the negative; being cruel in your assessment of yourself, your writing, other people and their writing, the situation and life itself; predicting the worst possible outcome of any endeavor and suggesting it's just easier to not try.

Denial And Excessive Optimism

Maintaining an unrealistically high opinion of the work and yourself, refusing to acknowledge or consider options for rewriting, rejecting any feedback that is not 100 percent praise, assuming that writing is and should be easy all the time, abandoning the writing anytime you're uncertain what to do, believing that "inspiration will strike" soon and there's no need to start worrying or stressing or trying until it does, assuming the writing will not need revising and there will be no rejection or setbacks, often followed by complete despair and abandoning the writing when these unrealistic hopes are unmet.

Overscheduling

Keeping yourself too busy to write by committing yourself to so many professional, personal, family and social meetings, appointments and obligations that there is no time left for writing, but thinking that the situation is temporary and being surprised that it's been weeks or months since you had time to write.

Underestimating Yourself

Committing yourself to writing projects that are safe, easy, boring and completely devoid of opportunities to write what you are passionate about, never submitting your work for publication or applying for contests and grants because you assume you're not good enough, enrolling in class after class after class and playing the perpetual student, not standing up for your writing and your right to write, letting other people's opinions count more than your own, and abandoning your vision.

Confusion or Forgetting

Feeling uncertain, hesitant and perplexed, having difficulty figuring things out, forgetting appointments with yourself or others, forgetting that every piece of writing is a puzzle and assuming that if you can't immediately see how it all fits together, you'll never solve it.

Sabotage

Any of the self-destructive activities the Saboteur takes against you (described in chapter eight), and failing to recognize resistance for what it is. Not all resistance is caused by the Saboteur; some resistance is appropriate. For example, it wasn't my Saboteur that paralyzed my legs on that cliff; that was my limbic system responding to real risk. But the Saboteur will use any and all forms of resistance against you whenever it can.

INSIDE THE WRITER'S BRAIN: YOUR CORTEX HAS LEFT THE BUILDING

You may recall from chapter two that when a person is stressed or threatened, the limbic system takes over and the cortex is unavailable. The limbic system will tend to avoid writing because that is the source of the anxiety that triggered the takeover. This, combined with the cortex's unavailability, is the neurological source of the common forms of resistance.

Losing normal access to your language centers causes the aphasia of writer's block and the sense of not knowing how to even start writing. Because the cortex is unavailable, you are more easily confused and forgetful. You can't quite remember what you were thinking about writing, and solutions to relatively simple problems elude you. When the cortex is offline, you are more distracted and may in fact seek out distractions to avoid facing the uncomfortable emotions that triggered the limbic system takeover—frustration, fear, anxiety, dread. Your ability to focus your attention and maintain the motivation you need to take action needed is also out of reach. Finally, since the ability to plan and predict outcomes is a function of the cortex, resistance can show up as overscheduling and excessive pessimism or optimism. Procrastination may arise in part because you can't access the cortex's executive functions of predicting future outcomes from present action and motivating yourself to take action.

That's Life; This Is Resistance

As tricky as it can be, it's crucial that we distinguish between resistance (in any of its variations) and the messiness of a creative life. We have to be able to recognize when the reason we aren't writing is not just a matter of circumstances that'll clear up eventually, but a matter of resistance that requires our attention.

For example, when the research piles up and your notes and drafts are getting so thick you can't find your desk, that's the writing life. When you have so many other non-writing appointments, projects and priorities that you can't find your way to your desk for weeks, that's resistance. When you have a medical procedure that requires mild anesthesia and you don't write that day, that's life. (When you're able to write about the discomforts of said procedure in a way that makes people laugh out loud, you're Dave Barry.) But when a routine appointment with your oral hygienist means you don't write for three days, that's resistance.

You can always find something to distract you or give you an excuse for not writing—that's the way life is. You're crazy-busy at your other job and that keeps you from your writing. Or work is slow and you're worried about losing the job that pays the mortgage, or you're unemployed and looking for a job, or you're a stay-at-home parent and that keeps you from your writing. Someone in your family or circle of friends gets seriously sick and you shift your schedule to support that person. Or ... or ... or. There's always something.

So how do you tell when you're truly resistant and when you're just adapting to life's curveballs? I keep it simple: if you're not writing when you say you're going to write, you are experiencing either a true emergency or some form of resistance. If you're calling the paramedics, police or fire department, on your way to the emergency room, or evacuating because of an impending natural disaster or invasion, it's a true emergency. If you're looking for the master shutoff for your electricity or water, it's a true emergency. Almost everything else is a form of resistance.

And as soon as your situation moves from acute to chronic— that is, as soon as you adapt to the emergency and it becomes the new normal—if you're not writing when you say you will, it's resistance. If your computer crashes, that might legitimately interrupt the day's Product Time. But if your computer crashed two days ago or it crashes frequently, it's time to show up for Product Time with a pad of paper or on a borrowed computer. If you can't sleep one night, you might feel too fuzzy-headed to focus on your writing. But as one of my coaching clients who was struggling with pregnancy-related insomnia declared, "It feels worse to not write, so I have to find a way to fit Product Time into this 'new normal.'"

A former coaching client, Laura G., had severe rheumatoid arthritis and a host of other painful and compromising health challenges that ultimately took her life. Yet she consistently found the time and strength to write. When she could no longer type, she learned to use voice-recognition software. When she was confined to her wheelchair, she had friends help her make her writing space chair-friendly. Each time her mobility and abilities declined, Laura found a way to adapt to the new normal that kept writing in her life. If Laura had that kind of courage, I think the rest of us can manage to show up for Product Time even if the kids are screaming in the other room, the cat is throwing up on the rug, or we're struggling with finding our rhythm again after a weeklong vacation break.

I'm not saying it's easy. But I am saying we can make it simple: either you're a) honoring your commitments, b) facing a true emergency or c) dealing with resistance. And you need to know which category you're in.

CHALLENGE: RECOGNIZE YOUR REALITY (AND SCHEDULE ACCORDINGLY)

I show up for at least fifteen minutes of Product Time 99 percent of the days I say I will, *and* I work through resistance to get there almost every day. If my calendar and my Product Time chart say I'm scheduled to start Product Time at 9:00 a.m. and I'm doing anything else at 9:00 a.m., I know I'm resisting my writing. I know my sleep routines, and I've already reviewed my calendar to determine that is it reasonable to show up for writing at 9:00 a.m. on that day (or I wouldn't have scheduled it at that time). So, short of being on my way to the emergency room, there is no explanation other than resistance. I make it easy for myself to recognize my resistance so I can quickly go through the four steps of Recognize, Relax, Respect and Redirect. I take these four steps nearly every day. Then I write. Because that's what I said I'd do.

If your calendar and Product Time chart say you're scheduled to start your Product Time at a particular time, but you consistently find yourself busy with other responsibilities and activities that truly must happen at that time, you need to acknowledge the reality that the schedule is not working for you. Scheduling Product Time when you honestly can't show up reinforces instead of resolving your resistance. It sets you up for failure.

For example, if you commit to Product Time at six in the morning, but you never get there because you can't get yourself out of bed at 5:00 a.m., you need to alter your schedule. If you're unwilling to go to bed earlier so you can get up at the time you think you should, or if you're simply not the kind of person who wakes up easily and well rested at that time, you need to move your Product Time to later in the morning or eliminate and/or postpone some of your other morning activities.

Review your schedule. Is it realistic? Is it reasonable to expect that you can consistently show up for Product Time at the times you've committed to? If not, change your schedule (this may require letting go of some activities that are less important to you than your writing). When your schedule for Product Time is realistic, you can easily recognize resistance: If you're not present for Product Time when you've scheduled yourself to be there, you're in resistance.

Why the Why Doesn't Matter

Many writers want to focus on figuring out why they're blocked and exactly which sling and arrow of outrageous fortune in their past is causing their current resistance. Sometimes knowing why can help you overcome the resistance. If Aimee, the French amnesiac, could remember why she didn't want to shake her doctor's hand, she could take action to make sure he didn't stick her with a pin again. If you know why you're resisting your writing, it may help you develop strategies to get around the block.

But—and I can't emphasize this enough—if you don't know, don't worry about it. Don't focus on the problem and fret over what caused it. It is not necessary to know why you're resistant to be able to respond effectively to the resistance. Overfocusing on the why can actually interfere with the what and how of taking the four steps that will move you past the resistance.

CHALLENGE: HOW DO YOU DO, HAVEN'T WE MET BEFORE?

In the How Do You Do? challenge in chapter two, you started a freewrite list of some of the ways you experience resistance. Review and refine that list to include the categories listed in this chapter. What kinds of things do you do and what does your inner voice say when you're resistant? What does it look and feel like when you experience:

- Writer's block
- Procrastination
- Postponing
- Distraction
- Perfectionism
- Hypercriticism and excessive pessimism
- Denial and excessive optimism
- Overscheduling
- Underestimating yourself
- Confusion and forgetfulness
- Sabotage

Which of these variations do you experience most often? Is there a predictable pattern in your resistance?

CHALLENGE: FIND THE MISSING LINK

Resistance often arises from a chain of "what-if/then . . ." statements. For example, "What if I sit down to write and remember something really painful or embarrassing? And if I remember something really painful, what if I break down and feel horrible? If I break down, I won't know what to do with my feelings. If I don't know what to do with my feelings, I'll be a mess. I'll have a nervous breakdown and have to take time off from work. If I take time off from work, I could lose my job. If I lose my job, I'll go bankrupt and lose my house and end up living on the streets."

Through some twist of illogic, sitting down to write means losing everything and living on the streets. No wonder you feel resistant and distract yourself with something else to do.

Your challenge is to follow the logic chain and find the missing links. What assumptions are you making that just don't hold up to reasonable scrutiny? And what reasonable action could you take if something unpleasant did happen?

For example, "Just because I start writing doesn't mean I'll remember something painful; I might remember wonderful things. If I do remember something painful, I'll still be okay. I can handle painful memories. Even if I break down and feel horrible, I won't always feel that way. Even if I didn't know what to do with my feelings, I'd get help before I had a nervous breakdown. And if

I did have a nervous breakdown, my friends and family would help me. My boss wouldn't fire me for having a mental illness, and even if I did lose my job, I'd get another one. Sitting down to write is not going to mean I lose everything."

As Dr. Susan Jeffers says in the classic *Feel the Fear and Do It Anyway*, the key is to know that whatever happens, you can handle it. You may not always like what happens when you face your fears, but you will figure out what to do.

STEP TWO:
RELAX INTO RESISTANCE

As soon as you recognize you're resisting your writing, you can immediately go to Step Two. Do not pass Go, do not collect $200, go immediately to relaxing.

Resistance means your limbic system has engaged the sympathetic nervous system's "fight-or-flight" or stress response system. If you recall from chapter two, the thalamus sends crude sensory information to the amygdala, which triggers the fear response and causes you to react to danger (like jumping away from a snake) almost instantly and without conscious thought. Meanwhile, your cortex takes longer to more accurately and completely process the sensory information, which it sends to the amygdala. From a survival standpoint, it's highly effective.

However, when you experience writing resistance, you are not actually facing an immediate, tangible threat (i.e., you are not trying to escape a predator, wildfire or other natural disaster). You don't need the lightning-fast reactions of your limbic system; you need the slower, more creative, and sophisticated thinking of your cortex. You need to get your amygdala out of the driver's seat and get your cortex reengaged. The best way to counteract the fear response is to relax.

This, however, is harder than it sounds. As Dr. Joseph LeDoux points out in *The Emotional Brain*, the connections from the amygdala to the cortex are more numerous and stronger than the connections from the cortex to the amygdala.[1] In effect, the amygdala talks more than it listens, and it's not keen on the idea of surrendering the driver's seat. Further compromising our ability to relax, the arousal system axons that the amygdala activates feed right back into the amygdala itself, creating "self-perpetuating, vicious cycles of emotional reactivity."[2]

According to LeDoux, this explains why our conscious thoughts are so easily invaded by emotions and why it's so difficult to concentrate on other things, like writing, when we're in an emotional state.[3] He writes, "Arousal helps lock you into the emotional state you are in [when arousal begins]. This can be very useful (you don't want to get distracted when you are in danger), but can also be an annoyance (once the fear system is turned on, it's hard to turn it off—this is the nature of anxiety.)"[4]

Still, the amygdala does receive information from the cortex and hippocampus that can dampen and eventually cancel the fear system's arousal; otherwise we'd be in a perpetual fear state. LeDoux points out that a sustained emotional experience can't be maintained without feedback from the body. As one researcher put it, it's hard to stay stressed when your body feels like Jell-O.

INSIDE THE WRITER'S BRAIN: TRIGGERING THE RELAXATION RESPONSE OR "JELL-O EFFECT"

Dr. Herbert Benson, known as the father of modern mind/body medicine and the founder of Harvard University's Mind/Body Medical Institute, was among the first in the medical community to recognize the negative impact of stress in the mid 1970s. In *Relaxation Revolution*, Benson updates his definition of the relaxation response as "the opposite of the 'fight-or-flight' or stress response. It is characterized by the following: decreased metabolism, heart rate, blood pressure, and rate of breathing; a decrease or 'calming' in brain activity; an increase in attention and decision-making functions of the brain; and changes in gene activity that are the opposite of those associated with stress."[5]

In other words, the relaxation response calms the body and the brain (by reducing activity in the sympathetic nervous system), thus bringing the cortex back online.

Benson's relaxation technique includes ten to fifteen minutes of repeating a focus word while sitting quietly, eyes closed, progressively relaxing the muscles in your body, breathing slowly and naturally, and assuming an accepting attitude when your attention drifts and returning to your focus without judgment. Research conducted by Dr. Gregg Jacobs at Harvard's Mind/Body Medical

Institute shows dramatic changes in brain waves after using this relaxation technique for just five minutes.[6]

INSIDE THE WRITER'S BRAIN: FOREVER STRESSED

The human fear system evolved to respond to immediate, life-threatening situations followed by longer periods of time when the relaxation response was dominant. We are not designed to respond to chronic stress. Cortisol and other stress hormones build up and devastate the body's immune system. The amygdala goes into overdrive, and the hippocampus loses its ability to inhibit the amygdala and serve as a sort of limbic system brake.

The more traumatic a single experience is, or the more constant and chronic ongoing stress is, the more the hippocampus is impaired. This damages conscious memory and severely reduces neurogenesis, the birth and growth of new neurons that occurs in the hippocampus. The hippocampus becomes Sandra Bullock driving the runaway bus in *Speed* and unable to apply the brakes.

This is why it's imperative that you have ongoing Self-care practices, like meditation, exercise, adequate sleep, time to focus (which provides relief from the chronic stress of attempting to multitask) and time to play. If you carry stress in your back, neck or other part of your body, get a professional full-body massage on a regular basis. Work with a movement therapist or bodyworker to correct any physical dysfunctions caused by chronic stress. For example, I've discovered that my carpal tunnel symptoms are actually referred pain from the tension I carry in my neck and shoulders when I'm stressed. Consult with medical professionals about any disorders that may be stress related. These practices will keep stress from becoming the dangerous norm it is for so many other Westerners.

Relaxing in the Now

Drawing on the findings of a host of researchers in a variety of fields, my experience and that of my students and clients, I offer you this smorgasbord of ways to relax in the moment:

Meditate

In addition to being part of your ongoing Self-care, meditation can help you relax in the moment. Five or ten minutes of conscious, intentional breathing can bring you back to calm. Or practice a few simple yoga postures (the Corpse is one of my favorites) or a few simple tai chi or qi gong movements.

Breathe and Count to Ten

My mom always told me to count to ten when I lost my temper. When I used to count as fast as I could through clenched jaws, it never worked. But if I take a deep breath in, hold it for a moment, then count "one" as I slowly exhale and repeat, it turns out Mom's right again.

Cool Down

According to *The Owner's Manual for the Brain*, "The cooler your brain is, the more relaxed you are. The warmer your brain, the more aroused you are (this arousal can be either limbic or cortical."[7] Limbic arousal is the undesired form of arousal that causes resistance; cortical arousal is desired because it is the source of focused attention. So when you want to relax, "chilling" is an apt metaphor. Interestingly, breathing through the nose cools the brain, which may be one reason deep breathing is so relaxing.

Exercise

Walking, running, cycling, swimming, cross-country skiing, or other intense, repetitive physical motion relieves stress and relaxes the body and brain. Aerobic exercise is best. This relaxation method is particularly effective for those whose stress response includes increased testosterone (which is present in both men and women) and accompanying feelings of "being on guard" or aggressive.[8]

Spend Five Minutes with Your Pet

Grooming, petting, stroking, or playing with a dog, cat or other companion animal is widely recognized as a way to relieve stress and increase feelings of well-being. Getting your cat off the keyboard or dog out of your lap when you're ready to return to writing might temporary challenge your newfound serenity, but the love and joy are worth the risk for me.

Practice Progressive Muscle Relaxation

Intentionally tighten the muscles in your feet, noticing the tension in your toes, in the arch and across the top of your feet, really feeling the tightness. When you're ready, let that tension go with a sigh. Take a moment to notice how good it feels to let your feet become more and more deeply relaxed. Continue intentionally tightening and relaxing different muscle groups in your body from your feet to your legs, hips and buttocks, stomach, back, chest, arms, neck and face. (To download a guided meditation leading you through this relaxation technique, visit http://www.rosannebane.com/main/relax.mp3.)

Pray On It

Invoking the Divine, using whatever name or phrase you prefer, can be a source of relief. Many religious traditions repeat certain words or phrases as part of prayer, and this repetition can have a dramatic calming effect on the brain.

Break It Up

Break your writing task into bite-size pieces. If you feel any anxiety, break the bite-size pieces into baby-size nibbles. Focus on doing one small thing, taking one miniature step at a time.

Blow Off Steam and Move On

Scream. Vent. Write a scathing entry in your journal. Rant to a friend. But limit this; don't let yourself vent or rant about the same situation more than two times. After that, you're revving yourself up and increasing stress. Express your frustration, anger, pain or fear fully, then let it go. Tear up the pages or give one final scream and be done. The metaphor "blow off steam" comes from the days when steam engines had pressure-relief valves to prevent the engines from building up so much steam that they exploded. The trick was to blow off enough steam to keep the engine safe, but not so much steam that the engine lost power. Hence the recommendation to limit venting to a specified amount of time and then let it go and move on.

Appreciate

Use this as a follow-up to blowing off steam or as a standalone relaxation technique. Identify (out loud or on the page) five good things that happened today, five things you're good at, and five things that make you happy. Start a gratitude journal and read previous entries or make a new entry when you need to relax.

Laugh

Laughter reduces heart rates and relaxes the body and brain. It's hard to stay tightly wound when you're genuinely belly laughing. Save cynical or sarcastic humor for when you're not trying to relax.

Massage

Give yourself a hand, arm and neck massage or a foot massage. Consider a chair massager.

Take a Mental Vacation

Imagine yourself in a place where you were relaxed and joyful. Visualize as many specific sensory details as you can. The meditation practice of visualization focuses attention and calms the brain. If you have difficulty remembering a previous experience with enough detail, simply study any object around you, then close your eyes and visualize the object with as much detail as you can.

Play a Musical Instrument, Sing or Listen to Music

Obviously, you'll want to play music you find soothing when you need to relax.

Immerse Yourself

Calm or gently moving water is inherently calming. Relax in a hot tub or hot shower. Float in a pool, lake or stream. Listen to sounds of ocean surf or a water fountain.

INSIDE THE WRITER'S BRAIN: SELF-MEDICATING VIA DISTRACTION

In *The Owner's Manual to the Brain*, Howard suggests we can take our minds off what is threatening or stressing us by reading, watching TV, listening to music or engaging in a hobby or craft. He writes, "As we take part in a totally absorbing pursuit, any activity in the posterior hypothalamus [an area of the brain that triggers the stress response in the sympathetic nervous system] moves to its forward area and to subsequent parasympathetic arousal [which triggers the relaxation response in the parasympathetic nervous system]."[9] In other words, doing something that engages you stops triggering the sympathetic nervous system's stress response and starts triggering the parasympathetic nervous system's relaxation response.

If distraction is one of the ways you experience resistance, you may have been unconsciously trying to calm yourself and inadvertently overcompensated with too much distraction. Distract yourself just long enough to relax, then move on to step three, Respect, and step four, Redirect.

WRITER'S APPLICATION: IT'S NO BIG DEAL

In *Art & Fear*, David Bayles and Ted Orland relate the story of a ceramics teacher who divided his class into two groups: those who would be graded on quantity (fifty pounds of pots earned an A, forty pounds of pots earned a B, etc.) and those who would be graded on quality (creating one perfect pot earned an A).[10] Guess which group did better. As you might expect, students who focused on producing one perfect pot rarely did. What's surprising is that students who were going for quantity without concerning themselves about whether the pottery they made was any good not only made lots of pots (thus earning the higher grades), they also created the pots of the highest quality.

Put your writing in perspective; you aren't doing brain surgery or rocket science. Stop worrying about writing something great today. Just write. If it's no big deal, it's easier to do.

CHALLENGE: CHANGE YOUR ENVIRONMENT

Examine your writing space with a discerning eye. You want this space to be relaxing enough to keep you calm and your cortex engaged, but not so soporific that your cortex disengages from lack of interest.

Optimize the visual elements of your space. You want colors, art and objects that interest and engage your brain without overwhelming you. Colors that are too intense may agitate you; colors that are too bland may put you to sleep. Too many objects become clutter that distracts and makes it impossible to focus; too few may feel sterile and impersonal.

Consider the physical elements in your writing space. For optimal brain performance, use natural lighting as much as possible and supplement with full-spectrum lights. Set up your chair, desk and computer ergonomically. There's no point in relaxing yourself with deep breathing, meditation or one of the other relaxation methods and then tensing up as soon as you sit down at your computer because the setup strains your body. Consider hiring a consultant to advise you; it's easy to get into bad habits and be unaware of the cumulative effect on your body and brain.

Select the sounds in your space to minimize any that distract or distress you. If you have a water fountain, make sure the hum of the motor doesn't overpower the soothing murmur of the water. Most people find natural sounds of rainstorms, ocean surf, birds, etc. soothing. Play classical or New Age music when you need to relax. Some writers—Stephen King is one notable example—love heavy rock while they write, but experiment to see what effect different types of music have on your mood. Some writers like the white noise of TV, talk radio or people talking in the background, but keep in mind that when you're stressed or experiencing resistance, the sounds that usually energize you could easily send you over the edge.

Be intentional about the smells in your writing space. As Proust suggests, smell is profoundly powerful in evoking memory. It also affects mood and arousal/relaxation. Smells that reduce stress and increase relaxation include lavender, chamomile, lemon, jasmine and cedar, cypress, spiced apple and heliotrope. Scents of eucalyptus, pine, clove, peppermint and basil make most people feel invigorated and refreshed, so although they're pleasant, they may not give you the relaxing effect you need when you're experiencing writing resistance.[11]

CHALLENGE: HURRY UP AND RELAX ALREADY!

If you've ever suffered through a night of insomnia, you know that feeling like you have to relax can actually be one of the most stressful experiences possible. Rather than giving you what could be a counterproductive challenge to "Relax!" I encourage you to list relaxation techniques that worked for you in the past. Make a second list of new-to-you relaxation techniques you might want to try sometime, but don't stress over it.

STEP THREE: RESPECT THE WISDOM OF THE RESISTANCE

Now that you've recognized your resistance and relaxed your cortex into the driver's seat, you have more options than just the three limbic system responses of freeze, fight or run away. But one option you don't want to exercise is ignoring the message from your limbic system and disregarding the resistance you felt. Recognizing and relaxing wasn't a mutiny; you don't need to throw your limbic system off the bus. You want a whole-brain solution that comes with getting your limbic system and cortex to cooperate.

The stories of Aimee, the French amnesiac whose implicit (unconscious) memory system was unimpaired and who therefore had every reason to be leery of shaking her doctor's hand even if she didn't know why (chapter two), and Lieutenant Commander Riley, who saved the lives of hundreds of sailors aboard the USS *Missouri* because he trusted his instincts and emotions (chapter seven), both illustrate that the limbic system has vital information the cortex can't perceive. But your limbic system doesn't have the language centers, so you can't articulate why you feel the way you do.

Trust that even if you don't know why you're resisting your writing, you still have some valid reasons to feel the way you do. This doesn't mean you simply give up and let your resistance push you away from your writing forever or even just for a day; it means that the only way to truly move forward is to respect your resistance. You must be willing to listen to your resistance to gain conscious awareness about what you need to move forward.

The Leap of No Faith

I jumped off the cliff because I didn't trust my resistance. What would have happened if I had? I might have walked away without jumping and never thought about it again. I might have regretted not jumping, and that regret could have given my Saboteur ammunition to use against me so that I ended up criticizing and berating myself and feeling diminished.

I disrespected my resistance by denigrating it, pooh-poohing it and dismissing it out of hand. I'm not sure what I would have done that day on the cliff if I had respected my resistance. If I knew then what I know now about how the brain works, I might have walked away without second-guessing myself. I would've known that my limbic system was giving me a strong message not to do that, and that my limbic system has its own wisdom, especially in matters of physical survival. I would've known that, even though other people can jump and not get hurt, that isn't my leap to take.

Or I might have assessed the risks better. I might have tried out my idea of yelling, "Oh, shiiiiiit!" while two or three other people jumped. I could have learned how long it would take to reach the water so that when I jumped, I wouldn't panic. Or I could have spent more time noticing my bodily reactions as I watched other people jumping.

What I did do was reach one those bullheaded, I'm-going-to-do-this-no-matter-what decisions that got me into trouble so often when I was in my twenties. I ignored my instincts and jumped. And sat on an inflatable doughnut for a week. In essence, saying, "Screw you!" to yourself and flinging yourself off a twenty-five-foot cliff is the ultimate example of disrespecting your resistance.

The Non-leap of Faith

Sometimes we don't jump because it's smart not to jump. We don't criticize ourselves for not jumping off highway bridges. Our fear pushes us away from true danger more often than we realize. We don't even know what danger we missed. You have a creepy feeling about a parking garage and decide to park elsewhere. Was there an assailant lurking inside that your intuition detected from clues your cortex couldn't detect? Or were you overreacting to the crime scene TV show you saw the night before? You'll never know.

Sometimes our anxiety or intuition keeps us safe and we need to respect that. We need to assess the situation as objectively as we can, understanding and appreciating the fact that our cortex cannot perceive nuances that the limbic system can perceive. Lieutenant Commander Riley was right to follow his intuition. Sometimes resistance is correct. In fact, more often than not, resistance is correct. It gives us information, and even if we can't decipher what message it's sending, we need to respect it.

Resistance is *not* Henny Penny screaming, "The sky is falling," all the time. Rather, resistance tells you something is off. Resistance makes you aware that there is a mismatch between what your cortex believes and perceives and what your limbic system believes and perceives. Sometimes not pushing past resistance into the scary parking garage or off the cliff is the smartest action.

But we cannot allow our resistance to stop us. Just because you don't jump off the cliff doesn't mean you're stuck up there for the rest of your life; you find another route back to the lake. Respecting your anxiety about a particular parking garage doesn't mean turning around and going home; you find another place to park. Or you ask for an escort to and from your car. You find creative solutions.

WRITER'S APPLICATION: R-E-S-P-E-C-T, FIND OUT WHAT IT MEANS TO ME

The next time you notice you are resistant to writing, relax and then ask yourself these questions as signs of respect:

- What do I need? Is there something I need before I can take this risk?
- What would truly reassure me?
- What's missing? Time, support, information, commitment from someone else?
- What am I really afraid of? Can I minimize the risk to acceptable levels? What would an acceptable level of risk look and feel like in this situation? What can I or someone else do to get to that acceptable level of risk?
- Is there something else I could do instead of this?
- If I assume there is some validity to my resistance, what specifically am I resisting and why?

Listen. Pay witness to your resistance. Freewrite with open acceptance. Assume your resistance has something of value to say.

Listening doesn't mean giving up on your writing; listening means finding out what's really in your way so you can respond in a way that allows you to move forward.

When you know what your resistance is saying, you're ready to take step four, Redirect.

CHALLENGE: WHAT'LL YA HAVE?

When you are NOT feeling resistant, interview your resistance in the second person the way you might interview a fictional character. Prepare your questions in advance. You might ask: "What do you need? What's missing? What unintended outcomes are you trying to avoid? What needs to happen before you'll move ahead?" Sit in one chair to ask a question out loud. Before you answer—aloud or in writing—move to a second chair and allow yourself to become your resistance (the way a writer or actor becomes a character). Be open to the possibility that your resistance has a different persona, different speech patterns or behaviors. Return to the first chair and your usual persona before asking the next question. You can record your interview if you wish, but the process alone will give you a great deal of insight.

If you prefer, you can work with a writing buddy. You interview your partner's resistance and your partner interviews your resistance.

STEP FOUR:
REDIRECT THE ENERGY
OF THE RESISTANCE

Redirection is simply changing the direction or focus of your attention. It may seem strange to say this at the end of a book all about writer's resistance, but you don't want to focus too much on your resistance. You need to understand resistance so you can recognize it, relax about it and respect it. Beyond that, you really don't need to dwell on it; you need to redirect your attention to the positive.

WRITER'S APPLICATION:
ACCENTUATE THE POSITIVE

According the principles of Appreciative Inquiry (AI), an organization development methodology based on decades of social science and developed by Dr. David Cooperrider of Case Western Reserve University, dwelling on your resistance will keep you stuck in that resistance. One of the primary tenets of AI is that we get more of what we focus our attention on. So organizations that see themselves as problem solvers get more problems to solve, while organizations that see themselves as leveraging their strengths get more strengths to leverage. AI asserts that the kinds of stories we tell about ourselves and the kinds of questions we ask about ourselves are essential. A question that focuses an individual or organization on bringing something positive out of past experience to make the future better is considered an appreciative inquiry.

Rather than feeling remorse about the time you've lost in resistance, consider the lessons you've gained from your resistance. Freewrite about what you have learned about yourself as a writer and a human being. What works well for you? What new habits and practices have you acquired to respond effectively to resistance? How will these new practices help you excel in the future?

All of the inquiries at the end of the chapters in this book were designed to be appreciative inquiries. But here are a few more to help you redirect your attention to the very best things about being a writer. Freewrite answers to these questions from time to time, or use them as conversation starters with other writers. Write or tell a partner about:

- The best thing you did for yourself as a writer this week.
- A time when you were really happy or excited about your writing process or the writing you produced. What made that time so satisfying? Was it what you were working on? How you were working? Who you were working with? Where you were working? How did you get into that particular groove?
- A challenge you overcame to make time for your writing. It might be getting yourself to a writing class. It might be locking yourself in the bathroom so you'd have ten minutes to yourself for writing. It might be turning your back on your messy house to go to a coffee shop to write. Focus not so much on the challenge, but on what you did to overcome the challenge and how it felt to make time for your writing.

- A time when someone praised or appreciated your writing. Be as specific as you can about what each person said that was positive. If you received feedback that was both positive and critical, ignore the criticism and focus on the praise and appreciation.
- A time when you were unsure what to do and then figured it out. If you can't remember a time when you wrestled with your writing, tell your partner about another puzzle or problem you solved. Focus on the contrast of how it felt to be uncertain or confused and how it felt to figure out the solution.
- Your strengths as a writer, both technical skills (e.g., "I write great dialogue") and process skills (e.g., "I'm good at making time to meditate before I write"). Keep in mind that once we've mastered something, we do it automatically and therefore lose awareness of it. For this inquiry, try to include both the strengths that you are consciously developing and the strengths you've mastered and don't usually think about ("I'm solid on English grammar." "I rarely use the passive voice.")

Smarter Than the Average Whale?

Redirection is a standard part of positive-reinforcement training used in outstanding programs that teach humans and other mammals, including dogs, dolphins, killer whales, etc., to perform amazing feats. You can take pride in being as trainable as a killer whale—all whales are highly intelligent and have complex brains, sophisticated social structures and a system of vocalizations that probably qualifies as language. You'll never be able to leap three times your body length out of a pool of water, but you can learn to write with ease and grace.

Short of outright torture, you cannot coerce a four-ton killer whale to do anything she/he doesn't want to do, just like you can't coerce a human being to do anything she/he doesn't want to do. One of the frustrations of resistance is the realization that you cannot coerce even your own self to do something.

Smart trainers realize this. They don't try to punish behaviors they don't want the trainee to engage in; they simply ignore the behavior. They use food or some other reward to redirect the trainee's attention and energy back to the task the trainer is asking for or to a new behavior. They stay alert for opportunities to reward positive behavior as soon and as often as possible.

When the trainer and trainee share language, the trainer can be more specific than merely ignoring the undesired behavior. But effective trainers don't dwell on what the trainee has done "wrong." In *Whale Done! The Power of Positive Relationships*, Kenneth Blanchard recommends business and other organizations apply this redirection response: "Describe the error or problem as soon as possible, clearly and without blame. Show its negative impact. If appropriate, take the blame for not making the task clear. Go over the task in detail and make sure it is clearly understood. Express your continuing trust and confidence in the person."[12]

Likewise, you want to identify the problem causing your writing resistance as soon as possible. Before you can do anything else, you need to express your trust and confidence in yourself by relaxing so that you change the brain state that caused the resistance. There is no need to blame yourself, but it can be helpful to clearly identify exactly what you're committing to do in the future and to redirect your energy and attention to taking action to honor that commitment.

Spontaneous Redirection

When you follow the first three steps—Recognize, Relax, and Respect—redirection often happens spontaneously and without conscious volition. Resistance holds tremendous energy, but it's trapped in the tug-of-war you're having with yourself. Taking the first three steps can release that energy as suddenly as when one team in a tug-of-war contest simply lets go.

When you truly respect your resistance, the solutions are fairly obvious. You see what you can do and start taking action. Many writers instinctively follow through on actions suggested by their answers to the questions in the previous "R-E-S-P-E-C-T, Find Out What It Means to Me" writer's application, but if you haven't already done so, that is a great place to start.

WRITER'S APPLICATION: R-E-S-P-E-C-T, PART TWO

Review the answers you wrote for part one of the R-E-S-P-E-C-T exercise and list the actions you can take to respond to the concern, issue or problem you identified. For example, if you realized you feel alone as a writer and need more support, you might join a writers' group, join an online forum, enlist a friend who also writes to be your email writing buddy, take a class, hire a writer who's published in your chosen genre to suggest revisions, hire an editor or coach, etc. Specifically, list the actions you can take to:

- Get what you need before you can take the risk
- Reassure yourself
- Make the time, enlist the support, gather the information and/or secure a commitment from someone else
- Work slowly and steadily through your fears
- Minimize the risk to acceptable levels
- Accomplish an alternative task that prepares you for the writing you want to do
- Take any other action that will reduce your resistance and move your writing forward

INQUIRY

"Who are my heroes of resistance?" (For example, two of my inspirations are civil rights leader Martin Luther King Jr. and women's suffrage leader Alice Paul.) "What did they resist and why did they want to replace those things? How did they work toward their goals? How can I follow their example?"

10

WHY IT MATTERS

Your Success Story

By now you've probably realized that resistance isn't something you get to solve once and then check off your list and never have to think about again. Resistance is and will be your constant companion. When you have days with little or no resistance, revel in them. But don't be surprised or disappointed when resistance returns. Learn to see resistance as a sign that you are challenging yourself to continue to grow as a writer and a person by venturing into unknown territory.

As you strengthen your habits around Process and Product Time and practice consistent Self-care, the intensity of your resistance will decrease and your capacity to move through it will increase. As you create your own writing rituals/routines and develop ways to record and reward your efforts, you'll find that resistance is less and less of an obstacle and more a minor, pesky fact of writing life. Moving past resistance into the flow of your writing will take just a little extra energy, like the kickoff it takes to go from standing still to riding a bike or from treading water to swimming. You won't mistake it for a sign that you should go away for a while or give up altogether.

Now that you understand what's happening in your brain, you can stop engaging in self-defeating behaviors like berating yourself or assuming you lack willpower or some other magical "something" that "successful writers" have and you don't. The writers whose success stories have appeared throughout this book achieved their success not because they were more talented, more disciplined or luckier than you. They had two things that, up until now, you haven't had: information about what writing resistance really is, and hundreds, even thousands of hours of experience. They applied their focus, energy and intention to consistently use the information in this book to create sustainable habits that led them around the writer's block and into the writing life they wanted. You can have that too, if you put in the time and attention.

And that's what really matters: continuing to show up and invest your time, attention and effort into your writing, no matter how big or small your resistance is on any given day.

INSIDE THE WRITER'S BRAIN: NO SHORTCUTS TO MASTERY

Chess masters see problems differently than novice players because masters actually look at the board differently. Research at the University of Tübingen, Germany, comparing differences in how experts and novices process information, shows that novices look at each piece individually, while experts direct their gaze at the center of a field composed of several pieces. Masters see the whole board (or section of the board) as a whole, a gestalt.[1]

Furthermore, functional MRI scans show that novice chess players use only certain areas (lateralized areas along the ventral and dorsal visual streams) in their brain's left hemisphere to identify chess pieces and the relationships between them. Chess experts, on the other hand, use both the left lateral areas and the corresponding areas in their right hemisphere as well.

The scans show no difference in how novices and experts identify geometric shapes, which indicates that chess experts are not innately blessed with better object-identification skills. They didn't start with a brain that processes information about chess pieces differently; they acquired those skills through practice. Lots and lots of practice. As Merim Bilalic, cognitive psychologist at the University of Tübingen and lead researcher in the study, observes, "There are no shortcuts to expertise."[2]

Based on these findings, Bilalic and his fellow researchers conclude that experts are not merely more efficient in how they process information (in their area of expertise), but that they use "qualitatively different cognitive processes which engage additional brain areas." They also conclude that this is probably a characteristic of all experts, not just chess masters.[3]

Although no one has researched neurological differences between expert writers and novice writers, I think it's safe to assume something similar goes on in our brains. In all probability, our ability to see a writing problem more holistically and solve it more creatively increases with the hours we log in Product Time. Our ability to recognize resistance for what it is and effectively resolve it also improves as we invest more time in our writing.

Another study comparing novice and expert players of shogi (a Japanese game similar to chess) showed that expert players activate areas in their brains that beginners never do and that intermediate players use only when they are familiar with the patterns involved. The experts engage their precuneus, where perception and high-level thinking occurs, and the caudate nucleus, an area of the brain involved with goal-directed behavior and forming habits.[4] The researchers were a little surprised by that, but I'm not. It's all about habits.

Habit Begets Mastery

The only way to achieve mastery in your writing is to practice. You have to show up and keep showing up day after day, no matter what.

In *Outliers*, Malcolm Gladwell cites examples from music, sports, science and business to define 10,000 hours as the amount of time we must invest to achieve mastery in any complex skill. If that seems daunting, consider that Daniel Pink defines mastery as a level of achievement we can get very close to, but never achieve completely.[5] In other words, no one ever gets completely there anyway, so don't worry about how far you have to go. Besides, no one knows exactly when the brain shifts to the more holistic and efficient expert mode.

The key is to know you're in this for the long haul. Writing is not easy. There are times when the words just flow and you get caught up in the joy of creating, but those times don't come without investing a lot of time in research, incubation, brainstorming and hours and hours of practice.

No matter how old or young you are, no matter whether you have an MFA or not, no matter how much or how little you've published, no matter how many or how few hours you can tally toward your mastery level as a writer, you need to keep practicing and developing your craft. You cannot expect immediate expertise or immediate success, but don't assume you have to log your ten thousandth hour before you're good enough to share your writing.

You can get pretty good at something in a few thousand hours. Writers can include at least some of the thousands of hours we've spent reading. The human brain is designed to acquire spoken language; no one has to teach a toddler the syntax rules or vocabulary words of the day. This tendency to unconsciously absorb language use is at play when we read. People who read a lot tend to be better writers, and those who read diversely tend to be more versatile as writers.

WRITER'S APPLICATION: 10,000 HOURS A QUARTER HOUR AT A TIME

Just as Lao-tzu said that "A journey of a thousand miles begins with a single step," your 10,000 hours to writing mastery began with your first sentence and it continues one quarter-hour at a time in your Fifteen Magic Minutes sessions.

Not every word you write matters, but the fact that you write every day does. David Bayles and Ted Orland point out in *Art & Fear*, "To you, and you alone, what matters is the process. . . . Your job is to learn to work on your work. . . . The function of the overwhelming majority of your artwork is simply to teach you how to make the small fraction of your artwork that soars."[6] Most of what you produce while you're pursuing mastery is valuable only because it takes you closer to mastery. Today you shovel dreck, and tomorrow you may well shovel dreck, and the day after that, because that's the only way to get to the good stuff hidden under all that dreck.

Keep going! Show up for regular Product Time sessions. Don't take your commitment past the Fifteen Magic Minutes limit, but start gradually stretching your capacity for longer target times so you can log more hours toward writing mastery. At first, an hour will feel like a long time, but as you grow, you'll be able to work for three or four hours, then five, then six. If you experience resistance to your expanding target times, think of it as an added bonus: not only are you developing writing mastery, you're logging time toward mastery in resolving resistance, too.

INSIDE THE WRITER'S BRAIN: DUELING NEURONS

The neurons you use for writing can and will be recruited for some other task if you don't keep them steadily employed. One reason it's vital to keep showing up for Product Time even when you aren't sure what to do is to make sure "competitive plasticity" is working for your writing, not against it.

In *The Brain That Changes Itself*, Doidge defines competitive plasticity as "an endless war of nerves going on inside each of our brains. If we stop exercising our mental skills, we do not just forget them: the brain map space for those skills is turned over to the skills we practice instead. If you ever ask yourself, 'How often must I practice French, or guitar, or math to keep on top of it?' you are asking a question about competitive plasticity."[7]

Achieving mastery may be a matter of allowing the skill being mastered to dominate a large brain map space. Mastery takes so long to acquire because it isn't just practicing physical skills or rote facts, which would involve a smaller brain map; it's deep understanding of the concepts, principles, background and history of the field, which requires a lot more neural territory.

Teaching Story: Feed the Right Wolf

Continuing to show up for your writing day after day matters not only because it brings you closer to mastery, it matters because honoring your commitments is the way you "feed the right wolf."

The Cherokee tell a story of a young man who was struggling with anger and aggression. An elder spoke to the young man, telling him his anger was understandable because each of us has two wolves inside us: a good, loving wolf and an evil, hateful wolf. The good wolf is loyal, brave, lives in harmony, provides for the pack, strives for justice and will fight only when it is the right thing to do. The evil wolf has no loyalty, acts without consideration for others, perpetrates injustice and attacks because it finds violent joy in anger, destruction and despair. The evil wolf attacks the good wolf all the time. But the two wolves are fairly well matched and neither can get rid of the other completely.

"So which wolf will win in the end?" the young man asked.

"The one you feed the most."

WRITER'S APPLICATION: MUZZLE THE SABOTEUR

We all carry two wolves—the Saboteur is another name for the evil wolf—and every action we take feeds one wolf or the other. Sometimes what you do (or don't do) fuels the evil wolf's attack on yourself; sometimes it fuels the evil wolf's attack on others. Usually, it's a small thing: You skip doing Process or Product Time for a day or two and somehow your habit gets sporadic. Or you lose touch with Self-care and eat a sweet roll at work or miss a workout because you're so busy. Or you stay up too late and, because you're cranky the next day, you swear at another driver, sending negative energy her/his way and wishing that person harm.

You also do little things that feed the good wolf. Every time you show up for Process, Self-care and Product Time, you feed the good wolf (and strengthen those neural pathways). Every time you grab a healthy snack or walk a flight of stairs instead of taking the elevator, you feed the good wolf. When you're in a good mood and give yourself enough time so you're not rushed and give another driver a break, you feed the good wolf. When the good wolf is strong, you honor your promises and do what you know is right.

It may seem that the situation determines which wolf will get more energy and attention. But that's a dangerous assumption that gives the Saboteur wolf an edge. Because every time you feed one wolf, you make it stronger. You make it more likely that you'll feed that wolf again.

The smallest morsel fuels the Saboteur and keeps it going for a long time. The evil wolf will steal food meant for the good wolf if it gets a chance, and it gets a chance anytime you're not crystal clear about your intention and fail to follow through on that intention with integrity.

If you let the Saboteur wolf push you away from your writing, it will not be satisfied and go away. It will demand to be fed again and again. Eventually it will push you away from something else you love. When you practice your habits with integrity, you refuse to feed the Saboteur wolf. This strengthens your ability not only to show up as a writer, but to show up as a human being and be of service and enjoy life.

INSIDE THE WRITER'S BRAIN: COMPETITIVE PLASTICITY IS THE SABOTEUR'S WORKSHOP

The Brain That Changes Itself offers insight into why the Saboteur has such a voracious metabolism: "Competitive plasticity also explains why our bad habits are so difficult to break or 'un-learn.' . . . [W]hen we learn a bad habit, it takes over a brain map, and each time we repeat it, it claims more control of that map and prevents the use of that space for 'good' habits. That is why 'unlearning' is often a lot harder than learning, and why early childhood education is so important—it's best to get it right early, before the 'bad habit' gets a competitive advantage."[8]

The more we allow the Saboteur to determine what action we take, the more control it has over a brain map and the harder it is to practice a good habit that feeds the right wolf. The Saboteur is an outrageous squatter that moves into brain map spaces when the good wolf is on vacation and then refuses to leave. When it comes to the Saboteur's ability to use competitive plasticity against you, possession is ten-tenths of the law.

CHALLENGE: WHY WRITE?

Feeding the right wolf and refusing to let the Saboteur push you around is one significant reason to write. But not everyone has to be a writer; there are plenty of ways to bring your creativity into the world. So why do you write? Why do other writers write? What's the point? (These are questions the Saboteur would love to keep rhetorical because they become so powerfully positive when you ask them as genuine questions.)

Freewrite for ten minutes answering the question, "Why write?" List all the reasons you and other writers spend time craft-ing words.

Then freewrite for another ten minutes listing all the people who benefit and how they benefit from what you have written or will write (your writing product) and from the fact that you write (your writing process).

You Owe It to Them; You Owe It to Yourself

If you decide writing is not for you, that the effort is not worth the benefits you and others receive from your writing, you can choose to hang up your writer's hat at any time without guilt or recrimination. Writing is not the only way to express your creativity. You may be writing only because you need to complete a specific project, like a thesis or dissertation. If you don't see yourself as a lifelong writer, in all likelihood you'll turn your energy and attention to the creative outlet that is your life's work when that required writing project is complete. I think you'll find that the three practices of Process, Self-care and Product Time and the tools in this book can be adapted and applied to your next endeavors.

But if you do see yourself as a writer, if you are willing to put in the effort to earn the benefits, you have the right and the responsibility to write. You owe it to yourself and everyone else on your list of people who benefit to show up for your writing. You and they deserve all the benefits your writing can bring. Remember that the next time you feel "selfish" about "taking time away" from your family, friends or community to write.

Pay It Forward

Think about all the writers and all the books, poems, essays, articles, song lyrics and so on that changed your life. Write or make a mental list of a few of the authors and manuscripts that influenced you. Then imagine how your life would have been smaller, poorer, less enlightened and joyful if those writers had decided their writing didn't matter. What if they had given up? What if they decided they weren't up to the task of putting in all those hours to achieve mastery?

Your struggles are not unique. Another writer has had every doubt, every distraction, every thought of "my little contribution won't matter" that you've had. Every writer faces resistance, endures rejection and indifference, and struggles with the confusion and frustration of the glimmering idea that they can't quite capture. Stanley Kunitz wrote, "The poem in the head is always perfect. Resistance begins when you try to convert it into language."[9] Kunitz didn't write that just for you; he wrote to all artists. You are not alone in the struggle, but if you give up trying, you will be alone with the unspoken beauty and meaning you could have shared with the world.

What is unique about you is your perspective, your voice and your vision. No one else has traveled through time and space on the same route you've taken, and no one else will combine bits and pieces of your experiences and intuition into a new, cohesive whole the way you will. If you don't tell the stories you have to tell (in fiction or nonfiction or poetry or song or whatever genre you work in), they will never be told.

Writers give people they don't know—people who might not even be alive when they're writing—a tremendous gift. The writers on your list, and countless others who inspired those writers, gave you a gift. If you've been given the desire to write, you have an obligation to pay it forward by making time for your writing and making the effort to become the best writer you can be.

Success Story: Love Matters

Aspiring novelist Kate L. had been hearing the call to write for years without knowing how to pay it forward. "I was the kid who made up stories in the confessional, wrote fake book reports and fake letters to Dear Abby. But I didn't know how to start. I used to literally poke holes in my notebook as a way of saying, 'Hey! I'm here. Anybody home?' I didn't know what to do with my need to tell stories, so it went underground." When Kate read the description for a writing class, she realized, "This is it!"

"It took me a looong time to connect the dots, forgive and trust myself, and admit that I want nothing less than an authentic life from here on out. I finally understand the mystic's advice to find what you love and do it."

Kate knows she doesn't dare let go of her writing again. "It doesn't matter that I'm shoveling dreck. It doesn't matter that I don't know what's what or who's who. It doesn't matter that I betrayed myself a thousand times. It doesn't matter that my Saboteur sometimes says, 'Who do you think you are? The world's going to hell in a handbasket and you think you're being "called" to write fiction?'"

What matters, Kate sees clearly now, is that she keeps showing up to scribble, poke holes in the page or answer questions. "I'm doing whatever I can to find a way into this novel. I'm letting myself love what I love."

Public and Personal Success

How will you let yourself love what you love? What needs to happen for you to feel satisfied and gratified about your writing? What does writing success mean to you?

Some writing you do just for yourself: your journal or diary, morning pages (à la Julia Cameron's *The Artist's Way*), miscellaneous freewrites, the entries you make to track your writing progress and, of course, your grocery lists and to-do lists and so on. This writing almost certainly will never be published, and that's just fine.

Some writing you prepare for an audience. It might be an audience of one person or a small group of people you know well. It might be for a larger audience you don't know personally. Some of this writing may be published; some may not. There are more publishing options than ever before, and in some ways it's easier than ever to be published. A quick look at the current *Writer's Market* will prove that there is a print magazine, trade journal or online outlet for just about any audience you can imagine, from mass market to mothers of adopted children to miniature horse breeders. There is no need to be shy about your desire to publish your writing, and every reason to believe you will publish if you're willing to put in the work necessary to make your writing worthy of publication and to find the audience looking for what you're writing.

Writing is only half the communication cycle; someone else reading and understanding or feeling what you want them to is the other half. Completing the cycle is essential to achieve many of the goals you listed when you wrote about why you write: to educate, to entertain, to influence people, to change the world, to leave a legacy, to encourage, to enlighten, even to get revenge or get paid. Publishing is a satisfying way to complete the cycle, but what is traditionally thought of as publishing is *not* the only way to complete the communication cycle.

"I think the word 'publication' trips people up," muses children's author Stephanie Watson, "because they think it only means having a big publishing company in New York choose you, invest money in you and make this printed thing that people will then buy. Publication means so much more now. Writers have so much more control. You can be a published author online in five minutes with a blog. You can self-publish books, which still holds a little stigma, but not as much as it did fifteen years ago because even established, published authors are choosing self-publishing as a way to have creative control. My least favorite part of being an author with a big-time publisher is that there are so many people who feel they should have a say in what your finished work is. And it's not necessarily in the best interests of the story or your writing style."

Stephanie recommends writers have a diversified portfolio. "I will always have my private writing, and I will always want to have writing out there in the world. I will always want to have some books with traditional publishers, and I will probably self-publish some projects. Every form has its advantages and drawbacks, so if one project is disappointing, you have other projects you can turn to."

You can post your writing on a blog or other social media. My sister-in-law gets great satisfaction from posting her poetry on Facebook and reading the responses her friends and readers give her. My cousin published a great blog about her adventures in refraining for a month from shopping or spending money she didn't absolutely have to spend. You can self-publish by hiring a company that will help you edit, proofread, design and print a couple hundred copies of your book, or format your manuscript as an e-book. Or you can prepare a document in the publishing software that probably came with your computer and take it to a print center like Kinko's, Office-Max or Office Depot to print one, ten or a hundred copies to distribute to friends and family. If you're so inclined, you can create book covers and interiors that are individual works of art. You can read at open mike night at your local coffee shop or literary center.

WRITER'S APPLICATION: EXPAND AND DIVERSIFY

To follow Stephanie Watson's advice about diversifying your writing portfolio, you need to expand your thinking about how you can share your writing. Start by freewriting what you think public success means for writers. Then challenge yourself to write for at least ten minutes more about what else success could mean for you. List as many ways as you can imagine of how you could satisfactorily complete the communication cycle.

Start a list of who your potential audiences might be, both in general (e.g., single moms of multiracial kids) and specific outlets (e.g., *Family Matters Parenting Magazine*). Keep adding to this list whenever a new audience idea occurs to you. Or if you get ideas by topic (e.g., "Wouldn't it be interesting to write about . . ."), make a list of topics and list multiple audiences for each topic. Ask yourself, "I'm interested in topic X; who else would be interested?"

When Audience Matters Too Much

Stephen King's ritual is to open his office door when he's revising as a way of inviting the world in and reminding himself to think about his readers. But when he's drafting, the door is shut; it's just him and the story. "The first draft—the All-Story Draft—should be written with no help (or interference) from anyone else," King advises in *On Writing*.[10]

There are times to pay close attention to your audience; how else can you hope to hold up your half of the communication cycle with any effectiveness if you're not thinking about your audience? And there are times to ignore what other people think so you can focus on your process.

Stephanie Watson observes, "It feels best when both those plates are spinning—when your process feels good and you're having fun writing and when you're getting some appreciation and validation from others. If you're getting lots of accolades, but you can't write new things because all that external stuff is clogging your brain, that feels awful. On the other hand, when my first book came out, I was so expectant and hopeful about the reviews, it was probably impossible for reality to line up exactly as I had envisioned. The disappointment interfered with my writing process because I felt that impending judgment about anything new I was writing."

Stephanie has learned the value of equanimity around other people's responses to her writing. "I decided to treat reviews of my second book a lot more lightly. I read them, but I purposefully didn't put much stock in them, whether they were positive, negative or neutral. The funny thing is that I got more positive reviews with my second book than I had with my first book, but none of it elated me and none of it bothered me very much. As a result, I was better able to focus on my work."

Choose Your First Audience Well

When you do open your office door to consider the needs and desires of your audience, you need to select your first readers carefully. You need allies you can count on to give you honest feedback when and how you're ready to receive it and in ways you can use to improve the writing.

Be sure you tell your allies where you want them to focus their attention and what level of feedback you're looking for. I firmly believe that all feedback should start with 1) appreciation and congratulations, then proceed through the following levels only when the writer is ready to receive that level of feedback for that piece of writing: 2) specifically what the reader found effective, 3) questions the reader might have, 4) where the reader thinks the writing could be more effective, and 5) suggestions for revising. How many of these levels of feedback you should ask for depends on how well developed the manuscript is. When the writing is fresh, level one and possibly level two are appropriate. The more mature the writing is, the more levels of feedback it can benefit from. Be sure your readers understand that all feedback should start with level one, proceed through the levels in order, and stop where you ask it to stop.

WRITER'S APPLICATION: WHO'S YOUR BUDDY?

A writing buddy will give you the kind of feedback you need and a whole lot more. Allies can give you encouragement, inspiration, ideas, suggestions, acknowledgment and validation. They can commiserate about the challenges of writing and celebrate the big milestones and all the little steps along the way. They can often spot your Saboteur's interference before you can.

Perhaps the most valuable thing your writing allies can do is to help you hold yourself accountable. Accountability can come from sending your buddy a quick voice mail or email message like, "I'm starting Product Time now." It might be a weekly check-in where you describe what you said you'd do for Process, Self-care and Product Time, what you actually did for the three practices, and how you feel about what you did.

The members of a Mastering the Writing Habit telecoaching class I taught are still emailing weekly check-ins to one another more than a year after the class finished. Their check-ins keep them on track and in touch as they congratulate and encourage each other. The Around the Writer's Block accountability groups available on my Facebook page, www.Facebook.com/AWBWriters Groups, are designed to give you similar support as a member of an online writers' community.

Can Your Partner Be Your Writing Buddy?

Be careful with what you expect from your spouse, life partner or other family member about how she/he supports you. Some partners are gracious enough to be great fans, energetic promoters, discerning readers and skilled editors all rolled into one, but that's a tremendous burden to ask your partner to carry, even if she/he is qualified to do all those things. Consider what your partner can realistically give you.

From your perspective, writing is an important part of who you are that you may have doubts about from time to time, so a partner who reflects your doubts or expresses disbelief about your capabilities can wound you deeply. But as a writer, you have to be able to step into another person's perspective; so do that with your partner. Does your partner see writing as a frivolous hobby that cuts into the time you could be spending with her/him? Is it an excuse to "get out of doing your share" of income generating or household chores? Is it a dangerous, misplaced pipe dream that will only end up disappointing you, so the kindest thing your partner can do is to keep reminding you not to get your hopes up too much? Is it a (either conscious or unconscious) painful reminder of your partner's own unfulfilled creative dreams and the chances she/he regrets not taking?

Start by explaining how and why writing is important to you and how everyone will benefit from finding ways to balance your desire and need to write with the desires and needs of everyone else in your family. Ask your partner and other immediate family members how they perceive your writing. Consider how you want to be supported and how your family is willing and able to support you. Expecting someone to give you something she/he doesn't have to give is a setup for disappointment and emotional turmoil.

Most important, make this a reciprocal, mutually beneficial and mutually agreed-to arrangement. That way you won't feel small, dependent or indebted every time your partner gives you support and your partner won't feel resentful or rejected every time you disappear into your writing.

You want to have reciprocal relationships with all your writing allies. Many writers hesitate to ask for support because we don't want to feel dependent or less-than. Or we're afraid to commit ourselves to some future, undefined obligation. This is why it is essential that we have reciprocal relationships with our allies and that we define those agreements in advance.

Whether you're enlisting allies from fellow writers/artists or from friends and family, I recommend you make copies of the Ally

Agreement Worksheet below and use them as a starting point in a discussion about how you can share support.

Ally Agreement Worksheet

I,_____ would like _____
_____
to be my writing ally. In this role, I would like _____
_____ to take the
following action: _____
_____.
I, _____, agree to be _____
_____'s
ally. I am willing to take the following action to support
_____'s
writing or other priorities: _____
_____.

Starting Over

The final thing that matters is that you remain willing to start over when you need to. Everyone drifts from their commitments at times, and the Saboteur will try to take advantage of that. Sometimes you need to change things up a bit: shift what you do for Process or Self-care or change the focus of your Product Time to a new idea that intrigues you. The willingness to start over, to begin again and again and again, feeds the right wolf.

"What separates artists from ex-artists," observe Bayles and Orland in *Art & Fear*, "is that those who challenge their fears, continue; those who don't, quit."[11]

Bayles and Orland distinguish between quitting and stopping, noting that stopping is a normal part of the creative process. You start a project, and you either complete it or you decide it's not worth pursuing further and you stop working on that project. Every writer returns again and again to the search for her/his next project. Quitting, on the other hand, happens just once. "Quitting means not starting again—and art is all about starting again," Bayles and Orland claim.[12]

Quitting is the decision to never try writing again. And as final as Bayles and Orland make that sound, you can unquit at any time. To start again, you have to be willing to be a beginner again. You have to be humble, which is to be teachable. You have to learn new ways to approach your writing without surrendering the momentum your habits and practices give you.

As I draft this chapter, the blizzard of February 2011 is smacking two-thirds of the United States, and my previously too-parochial Midwestern metaphor of winter driving now applies to enough of you to be worth sharing. Those of us who grow up in the Midwest (and the Northeast and the mountain states) learn how to drive in winter. We learn that after the plows go by and our cars are encased in snow, we dig out as much as we can, throw sand under the tires, get in, and rock our way out (and I don't mean turn the stereo up as high as it will go). We put the car in reverse and go back as far as we can, then shift gears and move forward as far as we can. With experience, we can feel the moment before the wheels are going to spin, and pause at that optimal point. We keep rocking back and forward, gaining an inch or two in each direction, until we just know we can keep moving forward. We can tell the wheels are spinning a little because the speedometer says eight or nine, and we know we're not going that fast, but we are moving forward, so we keep going because momentum is too precious to lose. And suddenly we're out of the drift and onto the plowed road.

What we don't do is sit in one place and spin the wheels. The friction from the tires melts the snow momentarily and then it freezes into ice. Spinning your wheels just digs a deeper, icy hole. This is where your Saboteur wants you—not writing and berating yourself for not writing, revving the emotional engine, but going nowhere. If you're not writing and you realize you feel bad about that (and you will because you're a writer), then do something. If that doesn't work, shift gears and try something else. You might make the tiniest progress, but its progress, so keep rocking!

The other thing we don't do in the Midwest is abandon our cars until spring. (I know; the planet would be better off if more of us did abandon our cars and use mass transit instead, but every metaphor has its limits.) We adapt. We apply new rules and tools. Giving up on your writing because you've hit a difficult patch is like running into a detour on your way home from work and deciding you'll just have to live in your car because your usual route is closed. (Or if you're a New Yorker, it's like deciding to live in a cab because it stalls out or the bridge is closed.) You don't abandon your home because you hit a detour, and when you're a writer, writing is your home.

It is so much harder to start over than it is to keep moving, so if you feel yourself slipping or notice your practices are not as consistent as you'd like them to be, shift gears and try something new before you quit. If you have quit and you're not happy with that decision, change it. Unquit by committing to a small step and taking it. Rock your way back into motion.

Success Story: Hope in the Face of Disappointment

Stephanie Watson has had her share of setbacks, but she refuses to let them stop her. She's learned how to keep driving.

"I feel so much hope working on something new," she says. "Even though it's never as perfect as you hope it will be, there is nothing like the high of playing around with a new idea that enchants you."

Stephanie points out that even in the midst of disappointment, sometimes things turn out better than we hope. "In 2009, after doing National Novel Writing Month and feeling burned out, I decided to write a picture book every day for a month. One of the ones I just tossed off ended up being picked up by Disney Hyperion by an editor I'd met at Scholastic. She liked the book and said she didn't want to change anything. And wasn't that nice to hear!"

When Stephanie's editor asked her who she'd like for an illustrator, Stephanie suggested a few illustrators early in their careers. When none of them panned out, her editor said, "I wonder if we should just ask Mary GrandPré." Mary GrandPré illustrated the

American editions of the Harry Potter books, as well as many other children's books. "I've always been a huge fan of her work," Stephanie recalls, "so of course I wanted her to illustrate my book. But she's such a superstar that I assumed that signing her was really unlikely.

"But she said yes! Mary GrandPré is illustrating my book *The Wee Hours* right now, and hopefully it will be published in 2012. When that type of thing happens, it gives me hope to keep writing, even in the face of the disappointments that come along with daily writing."

Keep It Small; Keep It Light; Keep It Up

To make your writing matter, you have to keep your writing no big deal. That you show up when you say you will is a big deal; what you do in that time and how "good or bad" what you write in that time is, is not.

Regular writing habits are vital, and you have to be in this for the long haul. You must be willing to invest time and effort to develop mastery in your chosen craft. But to be fully present to your writing on any given day, you have to surrender all expectations. Today's writing always has to be no big deal. Just show up and trust that something will happen.

To develop the habits and stamina you'll need, you need to keep the play in Process, the care in Self-care and the time in Product Time.

INQUIRY

"What does writing give me? What can I give my family, friends, community and the world through my writing? Why does my writing—both my practice and what I produce—matter?"

CHALLENGE: WRITE YOUR OWN ENDING

The trick to a happy ending is to know when to end the story. Fictional characters go through difficulties, struggles, setbacks and agony in the course of achieving their life's purpose in a novel, story or movie. Are those afflictions a tragic ending or part of the trials a hero must go through to earn the happy ending? You get to decide. As long as the story goes on, there is still hope for a happy ending. You can rewrite the ending to any story, even a published one, even your own story.

What's the end of your writing story going to be? Who do you want to be as a writer? What do you need to do to be that writer? What habits will sustain you in doing that? If you could write any- thing and you knew it would be successful, whatever success means for that project, what would you write? What else would you write?

If success means becoming the next Stephen King or J. K. Rowling, I can't make any guarantees. But if success means com- pleting a manuscript you're proud of that you can share with the world and receive some moderate recognition and financial rewards, I promise you will succeed *if* you're willing to work for it. So go write all those things you want to write. Live the writing life you want to live.

If I were writing this ending, I would encourage you to keep writing. Keep showing up for Process, Self-care and Product Time. Keep showing up for yourself, your readers, your family, friends, community. Keep showing up for life.

But you're writing this ending. So what are you going to do to have the writing life you want to have and to be the writer you want to be?

Please Tell Me Your Story

I'm eager to hear what you think and how you're doing with the three habits of Process, Product Time and Self-care and the other tools. Please post a comment on my Facebook page at www.Facebook.com/AroundTheWritersBlock, or on my blog at www.BaneOfYourResistance.com, or send an email to Rosanne @RosanneBane.com.

Please tell me what's working well for you and what, if anything, you're still struggling with. Do you respond to resistance differently now? Where are you improving? What success are you having with your writing? Do you have questions? What would you like more information about?

I promise to read all comments on my blog and respond to all emails. I'll provide short answers on Facebook and my blog, and I'll consider all your questions and comments as I write my next book. I'd be delighted to include you as one of the success stories in the next book!

APPENDIX:
FORMING A WRITER'S SUPPORT AND ACCOUNTABILITY GROUP (S&A GROUP)

You need plenty of support when you are practicing new behaviors. A group of powerful, trustworthy allies can make the difference between acquiring the new writing habits you want or not. Allies bring new information and insight. They bring new perspectives and possibilities. They add their skills and resources to the mix. They help you hold yourself accountable and honor your commitments because they're excited for you and because they want your support in holding themselves accountable to honoring their own commitments.

Yet many of us have difficulty getting the support we need. We don't know how to ask or what to ask for or who to ask. Sometimes we're afraid to ask because we asked the wrong person in the past and were disappointed. It can seem like a huge risk, but unless you are already getting all the writing support you need from the people you already know, you have to take the chance that someone you don't know yet can become a powerful and trustworthy support person. You can maximize your chances of forming a functional support group by selecting allies with a bit of care and forethought.

It is important that people in any writer's group have defined expectations about what the group is supposed to do for each other. Making a writer's group functional requires a blend of foresight (to bring the right people together), compromise and service (to extend yourself for others), fun (if you don't enjoy one another's company, why bother?), and the courage to be honest. It's worth the effort!

TWO TYPES OF WRITER'S GROUPS

Every writer's group is unique, but there are two basic types of writer's groups: critique groups and support groups. Both are valuable, and it's important to know what kind of group you're looking for. When most people think of a writer's group, they think of a writer's critique group where members read each other's manuscripts and give feedback on the writing. A support group is focused more on sustaining the process of writing than on evaluating the quality of any particular piece of writing. This isn't to say you can't get support from a critique group or that you can't get insightful feedback from a support group; it's a question of the group's primary purpose.

This appendix is designed to guide you in forming a support group to help you make the new writing habits of Process, Product

Time and Self-care sustainable. Writers do need feedback at times, but you can make substantial progress without a critique group; writers *always* need support and accountability.

FINDING SUPPORT AND ACCOUNTABILITY GROUPS VIA FACEBOOK

My Facebook page, www.Facebook.com/AWBWritersGroups, is set up to be a clearing house for writers looking for other writers who want to form Facebook groups that will function as support and accountability groups. You'll find information about how to create and work with Facebook groups at http://www.Facebook.com/help/groups.

You can use my page (www.Facebook.com/AWBWriters Groups) to post your name and who you'd like to form a support group with. Or go to this page to see the names of other writers who have posted their interest in forming a group. You can send a Friend Request and message via Facebook to people you might want to group with. After you've asked a few questions (see suggestions below) and decided you've got a good mix of people, you can create a Facebook group through your own Facebook pages.

My hope is that hundreds, even thousands of groups of 4 or 5 writers will form, so I need to keep my involvement in each group to a minimum. That's the why the AWBGroups page is a clearing house where you self-select each other and take the initiative to form your own circles.

I request that people who use this page understand the concepts of Process, Product Time and Self-care, either from reading this book or attending one of my Loft classes, but I can't guarantee this. So you might want to ask about this and a few other things before deciding who to include in your group.

WHO TO INCLUDE IN YOUR SUPPORT AND ACCOUNTABILITY (S&A) GROUP

I think it's important for writers in an S&A group to:

- Share common vocabulary and concepts (Process, Self-care, Product Time, Saboteur, tracking, rewards, rituals, etc.)
- Share a level of commitment (it can be frustrating for a writer expecting to typically honor 100 percent of her/his commitments to be in a group with writers who think meeting half or three-quarters of their commitments is acceptable)
- Agree on how often you want to officially check-in (I suggest weekly) and what to check-in about (see below)
- Agree on how often you intend to update your status (weekly check-ins only, weekly check-ins and daily progress reports, milestones reached, etc.)
- Agree on how much of your personal lives you want to share with each other (for example, do you want to know that a group member's sick child interfered with meeting commitments this week; there is no wrong answer, but having different, unspoken expectations about this can be a source of irritation)

- Respect each other and always refrain from judging any one in the group (including yourself)
- Root for each other's success

WEEKLY CHECK-INS

Start your check-in with a summary of your commitments to Process, Self-care and Product Time, what you actually did in each category, and what you're committing to doing in the coming week. If you set targets (beyond your commitment) for Product Time, include those too. One format you could use is provided in the table on the next page.

When you check in, state just the facts. No judgments, no excuses, no explanations, no long stories. Just the facts. Then write a brief statement about how you felt throughout the week. This might include some elaboration about why you felt the way you did, but keep the focus on how you felt. Focus on body sensations or emotions.

Avoid the tendency to slide into judgment or evaluation. "I feel like I did a good job" or "I don't think I did very well" are judgments. They are statements from your cortex that open the door for the Saboteur to starting talking trash.

"I feel happy, sad, frustrated, wistful, anxious, thrilled, engaged, intrigued, embarrassed, dissatisfied, disappointed" are statements of emotions. Remember, emotions are messages from the limbic system, which excels in noticing patterns and deviations from patterns, but doesn't have access to the language centers. Emotions are valid information.

	What I said I would do:	What I actually did:	What I commit to doing in the coming week:
Process	15 minutes 5x M-F coloring or working on a collage	15 minutes 3x on collage 15 minutes 2x coloring	15 minutes 5x M-F coloring or working on a collage
Self-care	30 minutes 5x meditation 30 minutes 5x exercise	30 minutes 5x mediation 30 minutes 3x exercise 45 minutes 2x exercise	30 minutes 5x meditation 30 minutes 5x exercise
Product Time	15 minutes 5x M-F	15 minutes 5x	15 minutes 5x M-F
Product Time Targets (stretch goals, not commitments)	2 hours Monday, 1 hour Tuesday, .5 hour Wednesday, 2 hours Friday	2.5 hours Monday, .5 hour Tuesday, 15 minutes Wednesday and Thursday, 2 hours Friday	1.5 hours 3x (probably on Monday, Wednesday and Friday)

For example, "On Monday, I felt satisfied and proud. Tuesday, I felt a little frustrated. Wednesday and Thursday I felt happy and relieved I managed to get in all my practices because they were such busy days. Friday, I felt good about a breakthrough on a plot problem I wrestled with on Tuesday. Overall, I feel satisfied and happy when I'm writing and frustrated with the way my work schedule gets in the way sometimes."

Use the information from your emotions to guide you in making commitments for the coming week. If you're feeling frustrated, do you need to change your commitments or change something else in your life? If you're feeling excited, do you want to increase your Product Time targets or stay with what's been a winning formula for you?

RESPONDING TO GROUP MEMBERS' CHECK-INS

Decide in advance how you want to respond to each other's check-ins. In one group I know, members send each other messages announcing what they did for the week and what they're committing to doing in the coming week. They then respond with messages that they are witnessing each other's commitments for the coming week. Some groups offer congratulations or words of encouragement.

Again, there is no wrong answer, but advance agreement reduces group friction. You may choose to modify how you respond to each other as your group gains history with each other and probably grows closer.

Your S&A group will benefit from discussing two questions in advance:

1. How you want to support each other (by hitting the Like button or adding comments like "Good for you" to a

check-in post or by adding comments or sending email messages with more details).

2. Whether or not you'll give each other advice (never, only when asked, whenever you see something the other person might not see) and if so, how you'll give advice (marked "Advice Alert" similar to "Spoiler Alert" or only as questions or in "you might want to think about . . ." terms or in straight out directives).

You need to find the balance between a) helping each other reframe your perceptions to see your progress in the best possible light so you stay positive about your ability to set and keep commitments without b) letting each off the hook by distorting the truth of what you said you'd do compared to what you actually did.

Be alert for the tendency to collude (either consciously or unconsciously) to underperform with easy excuses for yourself or offered to other group members as consolation or reassurance. Also be alert for the tendency to understate your efforts; undervaluing your effort or results is a symptom of Saboteur interference. It's easier to see the Saboteur in another member; one of the benefits of a support group is that they can tell you when you're being too hard on yourself.

GROUPS EVOLVE

All groups go through stages. One common perspective is that groups go through five stages:

- Forming: when the members first come together and most of the members' energy and attention is focused on how much they have in common and how optimistic they are about the group's potential success
- Storming: when the members start seeing each other's human frailties and the group's energy and attention pendulums to focusing on differences, conflicting interests and styles and opposing opinions about how the group should function
- Norming: when the members honestly and respectfully discuss and eventually reach consensus about the group's norms, standards, guidelines and goals
- Performing: when the group can devote its energy and attention to doing what it set out to do in the beginning
- Unforming: when the group either accomplishes its stated goals or dissolves by mutual consent for other reasons

Some groups are ongoing; some go through a fifth stage of unforming. A few rare groups can avoid storming altogether; some groups never get past storming and unform before they ever get to performing. Groups that intentionally focus their attention on norming as they are forming or shortly after forming can reduce the amount of storming they go through.

My hope is that considering the points and questions in the previous sections and making agreements about how you want your S&A group to function will get you to performing as quickly and painlessly as possible. But don't be surprised or disappointed if your group goes through storming at the outset or if later storming requires your group to revisit and possibly renegotiate your group norms. The strength of a group lies in its diversity and diversity means you will have differences of opinions and styles. Even the most functional groups will have some conflict. Experts in group dynamics recommend group members move toward conflict, rather than running away from it or denying it. The sooner you put the conflict on the table, the sooner you can resolve it.

Making any group without a formal recognized authority (like a boss or elected or appointed leader) functional is a challenge, but the rewards you'll get from your writer's group should make the effort worthwhile. If not, I suggest you take the courageous step of raising your concerns with the group. I don't suggest you "take your bat and ball and go home" for minor problems, but if you feel your group is no longer a fit for you or doesn't give you rewards commensurate with the effort you invest, you can respectfully end your association with the group and look for a new group.

Remember, a group of trustworthy allies of can give you the accountability and support you need to acquire the new writing habits you want.

ACKNOWLEDGMENTS

First and foremost, to my partner Claudia Bruber,

    I love you

    One, Two,

    Many, Lots,

    Now, Always and Forever.

You are the biggest fan of my life and I am the biggest fan of yours. Together, we make all important things possible, live our vision and purpose, and delight in a whole host of wonderful extra blessings. Thanks for helping me increase the activity in my left prefrontal lobe to become an optimist. Thanks for the strategic planning your frontal cortex does so much better than mine that made it possible for me to finish this book on time, on purpose and still in love with it, you and the world.

I owe a huge debt of gratitude to all the neurologists, brain scientists, researchers and science writers whose books, articles and findings I've referenced and to countless others who also dedicated their lives to science. Your years of research, hard work, intelligence, innovation and insight created astounding leaps in our understanding of the brain and human nature. You did the real work; I did my best to translate what you discovered and apply it to writers and the creative process. Any misinterpretations or misapplications are mine entirely; the credit for the science that was my raw material is all yours. A special thanks to Joseph LeDoux and Norman Doidge whose books *The Emotional Brain* and *The Brain That Changes Itself* were my inspiration and invitation to explore what a deeper understanding of the brain might do for writers.

Deepest thanks to Chris Mosley, who meant it when she said, "If you ever have anything you want the editors at Tarcher to see, send it to me and I'll pass it on," and who didn't blink when I replied, "Well, I do have this proposal I'm revising . . ." Your willingness to send my proposal on with an enthusiastic endorsement moved my book from potential to probable.

Good writing comes from rewriting, yet opportunities to work with editors who have time to guide writers through our rewrites are unfortunately becoming scarce. I am profoundly grateful to my editor Gaby Moss and to the leadership at Tarcher who have the wisdom to let editors like Gaby do what they do best. Thank you Gaby for asking questions that allowed to me see the places where the words I put on the page weren't what I intended or what the reader needed. You are an insightful and generous observer, advisor, collaborator, coach and advocate—in other words, you are a gifted editor. I'm blessed to receive the benefit of your gifts.

Thanks to Rolph Blythe for showing me and the other students in your Loft class how to transform the raw passion, research and insight in our rough drafts into polished and targeted book proposals that make acquisitions editors take notice. And thanks Rolph for introducing me to my agent Michelle Brower.

Thank you Michelle for shepherding me through the process, protecting my interests, and answering all my questions, even the naive ones, with respect, just the right touch of humor and professionalism. Every writer should have someone like you on her side!

Thank you to the Loft Literary Center, a shining beacon for literature and writing right smack dab in the Midwest, for all you do for writers. You are the wellspring of more great books, stories, poems, essays, screenplays and performance art than most people will ever realize. Thank you for the privilege and opportunity to be a Loft Teaching Artist for over twenty years, for giving me the freedom and encouragement to explore the ideas and practices that became this book.

Thank you to everyone who makes the Loft work: staff, board, my fellow teaching artists and Loft members. A special thanks to Brian Malloy, Jennifer Dodgson, Kurtis Scaletta, Edward McPherson, Mandy Leung, Vanessa Fuentes, Dara Syrkin, Kelly Ceynowa, Mary Lanham, Andrea Worth, Paulette Warren, Linda Greve and Jules Nyquist. A special thank-you to Mary Cummings who gave me my start as a Loft instructor and collaborated with me to create "Creative Process" as a legit class genre.

Thank you to all my Loft students for sharing your hopes and dreams, your challenges and triumphs with me. Thank you for being willing to pay attention to and talk about your writing process, your struggles with resistance, and what some of you thought was lack of discipline and some of you feared might be fatal flaws. Thank you for trying my weird ideas and for helping me craft and refine what I learned about the brain, motivation, psychology and physiology into practical applications for writers. Most of all, thank you for every day you show up and put in your time to share your insight, inspiration and perspective with others through your written words.

I owe a similar, but much deeper, debt of gratitude to my coaching clients who did everything my students did on a deeper, more personal and artistically/emotionally intimate level. I hope you learned from me some fraction of what I learned from you, and that our coaching gives you as much as you give me.

Specifically, I want to thank those students and coaching clients who were willing to share their struggles and success stories so honestly, courageously and articulately in this book: Lisa Bullard, Spike Carlson, Annette D., John Drozdal, Elizabeth Fletcher, Jacque Fletcher, Sheri Hildebrandt, Betsy Hodges, Katie Hoody, Kate Larkin, Ann Lonstein, Mary Maloney, Pam McAlister, Laska Nygaard, Gordy Paquette, Peter Pearson, Eileen Peterson, Pauline Peterson, Miriam Queensen, Laura Sommers, Julie Theobald, Sarah Tieck, Stephanie Watson and Jackie Werket. Special thanks to Jean Cook for writing "Synaptic Jazz" in celebration of the book contract finally arriving and for permission to include it here.

"Thank you" doesn't begin to say what I want to say to my family and friends. "I love you guys!" is too informal, but it comes closer. Thanks for being excited with and for me, thanks for understanding when I was unavailable because I was working on the book, thanks for being who you are and sharing life with me.

Big, big thanks with cherries on top to my mom Lois Walker and my sister Glendeen Bane for being delighted with me (instead of annoyed) when the emails for the book deal came through during our first annual Door County vacation. You made it so much fun to brainstorm book titles and cover art and to fantasize how great the book will be. Thank you for believing in me.

An introvert's inner circle is small, but mighty. Mighty thanks to Cathy Williams, Julie Theobald, Bob Paetznick, Jane Hensen, Dawn Cvengros and Melissa Brown. You always asked "What's going on with the book?" in the best way possible. You helped me see that "author" is a cool part of who I am, not something I just hope to be, and that it is just a part of who I am. "Friend" is too small a word for what you are to me.

Thanks to my "Writing Agents" writer's group: Jackie Werket, Jaime Benshoff, Jean Cook and Sheri Hildebrandt. You've seen the book through all its incarnations and permutations and despite all the shape-shifting, you always saw to the heart of it and reassured me it was worth incubating.

And finally, and most important, thank you to *you* who are reading these words. Writing is only half the communication cycle—thank you for completing this cycle and starting a new one with your own writing. If you are given the urge, inclination, desire, or even a passing, but recurring, thought that maybe you'd like to write, you are also given the right and the responsibility to write. Brenda Ueland wrote that every one of us is "talented, original and has something important to say." I believe that with all my heart.

A student once told me that she wondered if there was something wrong with her. "I must really not want to be a writer since I'm not writing," she confessed. I said that it seemed to me that if she really didn't want to be a writer, she wouldn't be taking the class. I promised her that the resistance she struggled with was not a sign that she should give up; on the contrary, the fact that she had even the smallest inclination to write in the face of that resistance was the sign that she should continue. Her resistance was a measure of how committed she was, how important writing is to her and how valuable it is to her and others that she find her way through the resistance. I'm happy to report that she found it.

I suspect you have similar feelings, which is why I heartily thank you for your willingness to share yourself through writing. I know how scary and confusing it is to want to write and at the same time not want to write or not be able to write. Thank you for your courage to explore how and why you both desire and resist writing. Thank you for your hope and faith that this book will help you figure how to get past the resistance. Please let me know how your journey unfolds (at www.Facebook.com/AroundtheWritersBlock).

NOTES

Chapter 1. Introduction

1. Daniel Coyle, *The Talent Code: Greatness Isn't Born. It's Grown. Here's How.* (New York: Bantam Books, 2009), 30–53.

Chapter 2. Why Is It So Hard to Write?

1. Joseph LeDoux, *The Emotional Brain: The Mysterious Underpinnings of Emotional Life* (New York: Touchstone, 1996), 105.

2. John Medina, *Brain Rules: 12 Principles for Surviving and Thriving at Work, Home and School* (Seattle: Pear Press, 2008), 40–43.

3. Pierce J. Howard, *The Owner's Manual for the Brain: Everyday Applications from Mind-Brain Research* (Austin, TX: Bard Press, 2006), 45–47.

4. LeDoux, *The Emotional Brain*, 161–67.

5. David Rapaport, *Organization and Pathology of Thought: Selected Sources* (New York: Columbia University Press, 1951), 68–71.

6. LeDoux, *The Emotional Brain*, 181.

7. Ibid.

8. David Rapaport, *Organization and Pathology of Thought*, 69.

9. Carl T. Hall, "Rethinking the Brain: Studies Show It's Wired for Change,"

San Francisco Chronicle, November 10, 2002, accessed August 23, 2011, from http://www.drugfreeadd.com/rethinkingbrain.pdf.

10. Jill Bolte Taylor, *My Stroke of Insight: A Brain Scientist's Personal Journey* (New York: Viking/Penguin, 2008) 111–12.

11. Sharon Begley, *Train Your Brain, Change Your Mind* (New York: Ballantine Books, 2007), 127–30.

12. Norman Doidge, *The Brain That Changes Itself: Stories of Personal Triumph from the Frontiers of Science* (New York: Penguin Books, 2007).

13. Ibid., 162–63.

14. Ibid.

15. Malcolm Gladwell, *Outliers: The Story of Success* (New York: Little Brown), 39–42.

Chapter 3. Habit One: Process

1. Dorothea Brande, *Becoming a Writer* (New York: J. P. Tarcher, 1981), 72.

2. Brenda Ueland, *If You Want to Write: A Book about Art, Independence and Spirit* (St. Paul, MN: Graywolf Press, 1987), 32.

3. "31 Ways to Get Smarter in 2012," *Newsweek*, January 9, 2012, 33.

4. Gwendolyn Bounds, "How Handwriting Trains the Brain," *Wall Street Journal*, October 5, 2010, accessed on January 25, 2012, from http://online.wsj.com/article/SB1000142405274870463150457553193275492251 8.html.

5. Alexander Alter, "How to Write a Great Novel," *Wall Street Journal*, November 13, 2009, accessed on January 25, 2012, from http://online.wsj.com/article/SB10001424052748703740004574513463106012106.html.

6. Begley, "Buff Your Brain," 30.

7. Sue Ramsden, Fiona M. Richardson, Goulven Josee, Michael S. C. Thomas, Caroline Ellis, Clare Shakeshaft, Mohamed L. Seghier, and Cathy J. Price, "Verbal and Non-Verbal Intelligence Changes in the Teenage Brain," *Nature* 479, 113–16.

8. Taylor, *My Stroke of Insight*.

9. Ibid., 137–45.

10. Ibid., 140.

11. Ibid.
12. Anna Wise, *The High-Performance Mind: Mastering Brainwaves for Insight, Healing and Creativity* (New York: Tarcher/Putnam, 1995), 2–12.
13. Howard, *The Owner's Manual for the Brain*, 58–59.
14. Wise, *The High-Performance Mind*, 158.
15. Howard, *The Owner's Manual for the Brain*, 617.

Chapter 4. Habit Two: Product Time

1. Norman Mailer, *The Spooky Art: Some Thoughts on Writing* (New York: Random House, 2003), 142.
2. Betty Edwards, *Drawing on the Artist Within* (New York: Fireside, 1986), 2–47.
3. Rosanne Bane, *Dancing in the Dragon's Den: Rekindling the Creative Fire in Your Shadow* (York Beach, ME: Nicolas Hays, 1999), 215–19.
4. Mihaly Csikszentmihalyi, *Flow: The Psychology of Optimal Experience* (New York: Harper, 1990), 1–22.
5. Doidge, *The Brain That Changes Itself*, 63.
6. Coyle, *The Talent Code*, 30–53.

Chapter 5. Habit Three: Self-care

1. Matt Richtel, "Your Brain on Computers: Digital Devices Deprive Brain of Needed Downtime," *New York Times*, August 24, 2010, accessed on August 30, 2010, from http://www.nytimes.com/2010/08/25/technology/25brain.html?pagewanted=1&_r=1&ref=your_brain_on_computers.
2. Medina, *Brain Rules*, 163.
3. Howard, *The Owner's Manual for the Brain*, 193, 204–7.
4. Ibid., 190.
5. Ibid., 193.
6. Medina, *Brain Rules*, 152–53.
7. Howard, *The Owner's Manual for the Brain*, 193.
8. John J. Ratey, *Spark: The Revolutionary New Science of Exercise and the Brain* (New York: Little, Brown, 2008), 3.
9. Ibid., 66.

10. Ibid., 40.

11. Ibid., 51–53.

12. Begley, *Train Your Mind, Change Your Brain*, 68–69.

13. Ratey, *Spark*, 58–61.

14. Medina, *Brain Rules*, 16–17.

15. Ratey, *Spark*, 121–22.

16. Howard, *The Owner's Manual for the Brain*, 56.

17. Ratey, *Spark*, 102.

18. Ibid., 70.

19. Medina, *Brain Rules*, 15.

20. Ratey, *Spark*, 55–56, 138.

21. Ibid., 55–56.

22. Ibid., 53–54.

23. "Exercise Outdoors Brings Even More Benefits," accessed August 24, 2010, from http://www.elements4health.com/excercise-outdoors-brings-even-more-benefits.html.

24. Robert Olen Butler, *From Where You Dream: The Process of Writing Fiction* (New York: Grove Press, 2005), 31.

25. Naomi Epel, *Writers Dreaming* (New York: Carol Southern Books, 1993), 44.

26. Brandon Keim, "Digital Overload Is Frying Our Brains," *Wired Science*, February 6, 2009, accessed May 12, 2011, from http://www.wired.com/wiredscience/2009/02/attentionlost/.

27. Maggie Jackson, *Distracted: The Erosion of Attention and the Coming Dark Age* (New York: Prometheus Books, 2008), 93.

28. Medina, *Brain Rules*, 84–88.

29. Ibid., 87.

30. "Media Multitaskers Pay Mental Price, Stanford Study Shows," accessed August 24, 2011, from http://news.stanford.edu/pr/2009/multitask-research-release-082409.html.

31. Ibid.

32. Matt Richtel, "Your Brain on Computers: Addicted to Technology and Paying a Price," *New York Times*, June 6, 2010, accessed August 31, 2010, from http://www.nytimes.com/2010/06/07/technology/07brain.html?ref=your_brain_on_computers.

33. Ibid.

34. Ibid.

35. Begley, *Train Your Mind, Change Your Brain*, 212–42.

36. Mihaly Csikszentmihalyi, *Creativity: Flow and the Psychology of Discovery and Invention* (New York: HarperCollins, 1996), 112–13.

37. Begley, *Train Your Mind, Change Your Brain*, 234.

38. Ibid., 213, 235.

39. Judith Horstman, *The Scientific American Brave New Brain* (San Francisco: Jossey-Bass, 2010), 31.

40. Ibid., 34.

41. Begley, *Train Your Mind, Change Your Brain*, 234–35.

42. Ibid., 242.

43. Richard J. Davidson, John Kabat-Zinn, Jessica Schumacher, Melissa Rosenkranz, Daniel Muller, Saki F. Santorelli, Ferris Urbanowski, Anne Harrington, Katherine Bonus, and John F. Sheridan, "Alterations in Brain and Immune Function Produced by Mindfulness Meditation," *Psychosomatic Medicine*, 65 (2003): 564–70.

44. Thérèse Jacobs-Stewart, *Paths Are Made By Walking: Practical Steps for Attaining Serenity* (New York: Warner Books, 2003), 18.

45. Begley, *Train Your Mind, Change Your Brain*, 225.

46. Hortsman, *The Scientific American Brave New Brain*, 32–33.

47. Davidson, et al., "Alterations in Brain and Immune Function Produced by Mindfulness Meditation," 564–70.

48. Stuart Brown, *Play: How It Shapes the Brain, Opens the Imagination and Invigorates the Soul* (New York: Avery/Penguin Books, 2009), 17.

49. Horstman, *The Scientific American Brave New Brain*, 66.

50. Doidge, *The Brain That Changes Itself*, 256.

51. Brown, *Play*, 33–34.

52. Ibid., 41.

53. Ibid., 33.

54. Ibid., 43.

55. Ibid., 58–59, 71.

56. Ibid., 44.

57. Ibid., 61–62.

58. Horstman, *The Scientific American Brave New Brain*, 66–67.

Chapter 6. Rituals and Routines

1. Ralph Keyes, *The Courage to Write: How Writers Transcend Fear* (New York: Holt, 1995), 136–37.
2. Ibid., 140.
3. Ibid.
4. Twyla Tharp, *The Creative Habit: Learn It and Live It for Life* (New York: Simon & Schuster, 2003), 15.
5. Butler, *From Where You Dream*, 22.
6. Medina, *Brain Rules*, 213.
7. Ibid., 213, 215–16.
8. Coyle, *The Talent Code*, 44–45.

Chapter 7. Record and Reward

1. Jeffrey M. Schwartz and Sharon Begley, *The Mind and The Brain: Neuroplasticity and the Power of Mental Force* (New York: Harper, 2002), 209–12.
2. Ibid., 338.
3. "Want to Lose Weight? Keep a Food Diary," accessed October 6, 2010, from http://www.medicalnewstoday.com/articles/114298.php.
4. Csikszentmihalyi, *Creativity*, 115–16.
5. Jonah Lehrer, *How We Decide* (New York: Houghton Mifflin Harcourt, 2009), 30–34, 55–56.
6. Doidge, *The Brain That Changes Itself*, 71, 107, 113.
7. Lehrer, *How We Decide*, 36–38.
8. Daniel H. Pink, *Drive: The Surprising Truth about What Motivates Us* (New York: Riverhead/Penguin, 2009), 34–69.
9. Ibid., 39, quoting Edward L. Deci, Richard M. Ryan, and Richard Koestner, "A Meta-Analytic Review of Experiments Examining the Effects of Extrinsic Rewards on Intrinsic Motivation", *Psychological Bulletin* 125, no. 6 (1999), 659.
10. Pink, *Drive*, 44–45.
11. Howard, *The Owner's Manual for the Brain*, 613.
12. Pink, *Drive*, 46.
13. Ibid., 62.
14. Lehrer, *How We Decide*, 52–53.

15. Doidge, *The Brain That Changes Itself*, 147.
16. Ibid., 143.
17. Lehrer, *How We Decide*, 60.
18. Ibid., 184.

Chapter 8. Why Is It So Hard to Write, Revisited

1. Caroline Myss, *Sacred Contracts: Awakening Your Divine Potential* (New York: Harmony Books, 2001), 122.
2. John Darling, "The Ironic Gifts of the Predator Archetype," *New Connexion*, July/August 2006, accessed November 22, 2010, from http://newconnexion.net/articles/index.cfm/2006/07/Predator_Archetype.html.
3. Taylor, *My Stroke of Insight*, 152.
4. Ibid.
5. Ibid.
6. Ibid., 153–54.
7. Jacquelyn B. Fletcher, "Squelch Your Inner Censor," *Writer's Digest*, November 2005, 36–37.
8. Doidge, *The Brain That Changes Itself*, 168.
9. Schwartz and Begley, *The Mind and the Brain*, 55.
10. Ibid., 55.
11. Ibid., 60–68.
12. Doidge, *The Brain That Changes Itself*, 165.
13. Schwartz and Begley, *The Mind and the Brain*, 78–82.
14. Ibid., 82.

Chapter 9. Four Steps to Resolving Resistance

1. LeDoux, *The Emotional Brain*, 284.
2. Ibid., 290.
3. Ibid., 265.
4. Ibid., 289.
5. Herbert Benson, *The Relaxation Revolution: The Science and Genetics of Mind Body Healing* (New York: Scribner, 2010), 56.
6. Howard, *The Owner's Manual for the Brain*, 349.

7. Ibid., 730.

8. Ibid., 821, 828.

9. Ibid., 821.

10. David Bayles and Ted Orland, *Art & Fear: Observations on the Perils (and Rewards) of Artmaking* (Santa Cruz, CA: Image Continuum, 1993), 29.

11. Howard, *The Owner's Manual for the Brain*, 723.

12. Kenneth Blanchard, *Whale Done! The Power of Positive Relationships* (New York: Free Press, 2002), 34.

Chapter 10. Why It Matters

1. Dylan Loeb McClain, "Harnessing the Brain's Right Hemisphere to Capture Many Kings," *New York Times*, January 24, 2011, accessed January 28, 2011, from http://www.nytimes.com/2011/01/25/science/25chess.html?_r=1&ref=science.

2. Ibid.

3. Merim Bilalic, Andrea Kiesel, Carsten Pohl, Michael Erb, and Wolfgang Grodd, "It Takes Two: Skilled Recognition of Objects Engages Lateral Areas in Both Hemispheres," *PLoS ONE* 6(1), accessed January 28, 2011, from http://www.plosone.org/article/info%3Adoi%2F10.1371%2Fjournal.pone.0016202.

4. McClain, "Harnessing the Brain's Right Hemisphere to Capture Many Kings."

5. Pink, *Drive*, 126–27.

6. Bayles and Orland, *Art & Fear*, 5.

7. Doidge, *The Brain That Changes Itself*, 59.

8. Ibid., 60.

9. Bayles and Orland, *Art & Fear*, 17.

10. Stephen King, *On Writing: A Memoir of the Craft* (New York: Scribner, 2000), 209.

11. Bayles and Orland, *Art & Fear*, 14.

12. Ibid., 10.

INDEX